HIGH-RESOLUTION NEUROIMAGING - BASIC PHYSICAL PRINCIPLES AND CLINICAL APPLICATIONS

Edited by **Ahmet Mesrur Halefoğlu**

High-Resolution Neuroimaging - Basic Physical Principles and Clinical Applications
http://dx.doi.org/10.5772/intechopen.68268
Edited by Ahmet Mesrur Halefoğlu

Contributors

Yukifumi Monden, Ippeita Dan, Masako Nagashima, Takahiro Ikeda, Takanori Yamagata, Yasushi Kyutoku, Haruka Dan, Nicole Schubert, Markus Axer, Uwe Pietrzyk, Katrin Amunts, Neha Mathur, Shruti Mathur, Divya Mathur, Dr. Yogesh Kumar Meena, Hanafy Ali, Vinicius Carvalho Rispoli, Joao Carvalho, Cristiano Miosso, Fabiano Soares, A.R.Kavitha Balaji, Chellamuthu Chinna Gounder, Jianfeng Zheng, Ran Guo, Kenya Murase, Sunao Shoji

Published by InTech

Janeza Trdine 9, 51000 Rijeka, Croatia

Publishing Process Manager Marijana Francetic
Technical Editor SPi Global
Cover InTech Design team

First published March, 2018
Printed in Croatia
Legal deposit, Croatia: National and University Library in Zagreb

Additional hard copies can be obtained from orders@intechopen.com

High-Resolution Neuroimaging - Basic Physical Principles and Clinical Applications, Edited by Ahmet Mesrur Halefoğlu
p. cm.
Print ISBN 978-953-51-3865-5
Online ISBN 978-953-51-3866-2

For EU product safety concerns:
IN TECH d.o.o., Prolaz Marije Krucifikse Kozulić 3, 51000 Rijeka, Croatia,
info@intechopen.com or visit our website at intechopen.com.

Meet the editor

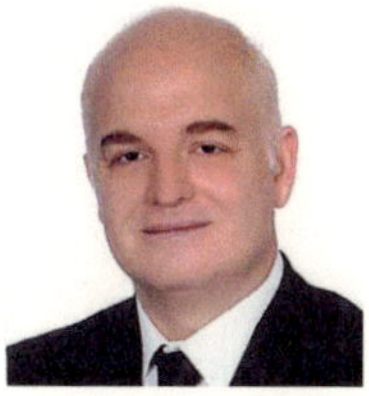

Dr. Ahmet Mesrur Halefoğlu is currently working as a resident specialist of Radiology and professor at Sisli Etfal Training and Research Hospital, Istanbul, Turkey. He has completed Antakya High School at Antakya, Hatay, Turkey, with honor degree and has graduated from Istanbul University Cerrahpaşa School of Medicine in 1986, Istanbul, Turkey. He completed his residency between 1992 and 1997 at Sisli Etfal Training and Research Hospital, Istanbul, Turkey. He served as postdoctoral research fellow at Johns Hopkins Hospital, Baltimore, MD, USA, between 1998 and 1999. He has also been a research observer at Johns Hopkins Hospital in 2002 and 2004. He is mostly dealing with research fields in body imaging and neuroradiology with multidetector computed tomography and high-resolution magnetic resonance imaging. He has more than 50 high-impact-factor publications and has written 3 book chapters. He is a member of Turkish Society of Radiology and European Society of Radiology.

Contents

Preface

It is my pleasure to introduce the book entitled *High-Resolution Neuroimaging - Basic Physical Principles and Clinical Applications*. The advent of MRI has provided noninvasive visualization of the human body, including the brain and spinal cord, in a high-quality manner.

MRI has the capability of producing more detailed images compared to other cross-sectional images, namely, ultrasound and computed tomography. This modality is based on the principle of magnetic excitation of the hydrogen nuclei, which are found throughout the human body, by using strong magnetic fields. This can be achieved by applying RF pulses and then measuring the emitted signal.

MRI is regarded as an essential modality with excellent soft tissue contrast resolution in the diagnosis of pathological conditions, predicting the prognosis and the planning of treatment strategies in patients with a variety of neurological disorders.

During the recent years, there have been major breakthroughs in MRI due to developments in scanner technology and pulse sequencing. These important achievements have led to remarkable improvements in neuroimaging and advanced techniques, including diffusion imaging, diffusion tensor imaging, perfusion imaging, magnetic resonance spectroscopy, and functional MRI. These advanced neuroimaging techniques have enabled us to achieve invaluable insights into tissue microstructure, microvasculature, metabolism, and brain connectivity.

The aim of this book is to introduce some of these advanced high-resolution neuroimaging techniques and also to demonstrate their basic physical principles and clinical applications in various neurological disorders.

Ahmet Mesrur Halefoğlu , MD
Department of Radiology
Sisli Hamidiye Etfal Training and Research Hospital
Istanbul, Turkey

Section 1

Health Sciences

Chapter 1

fNIRS-Based Clinical Assessment of ADHD Children

Yukifumi Monden, Masako Nagashima,
Haruka Dan, Takahiro Ikeda, Yasushi Kyutoku,
Takanori Yamagata and Ippeita Dan

Additional information is available at the end of the chapter

http://dx.doi.org/10.5772/intechopen.71835

Abstract

While a growing body of neurocognitive research has explored the neural substrates associated with attention deficit hyperactive disorder (ADHD), an objective biomarker for diagnosis has not been established. The advent of functional near-infrared spectroscopy (fNIRS), which is a noninvasive and unrestrictive method of functional neuroimaging, raised the possibility of introducing functional neuroimaging diagnosis for young ADHD children. In search of a stable and clinically applicable biological marker, here in this chapter, we first discuss a plausible solution to enable the objective monitoring of the acute effects of ADHD medications at the group level. Subsequently, we discuss our successful visualization of differential neural substrates between ADHD and healthy control children for inhibitory control at the individual level, which reached an optimized classification parameter with a value of 85% and a sensitivity of 90%. These findings led us to postulate that fNIRS-based examination would allow the identification of an objective neuro-functional biomarker to diagnose and determine the appropriate treatment for ADHD children. We believe that such a novel technical application would evoke wide interest from neuroimaging researchers.

Keywords: developmental syndromes, optical topography, response inhibition, autism, discrimination analysis

1. Introduction

Noninvasive functional neuroimaging has been introduced as a promising approach, in combination with psychological tests, to clinical diagnosis. Functional near-infrared spectroscopy (fNIRS) is an increasingly popular neuroimaging technique which noninvasively monitors human brain activation patterns, utilizing the tight coupling between neural activity and regional cerebral hemodynamic responses, which has a high affinity with the study of developing brains (reviewed in, for example, [1–5]).

fNIRS has distinct advantages in its compactness, tolerance to body motion, affordable price, and accessibility [2, 6–11]. These advantages allow fNIRS to be contrasted with conventional imaging modalities such as functional magnetic resonance imaging (fMRI), single photon emission computed tomography (SPECT), positron emission tomography (PET), and magnetoencephalography (MEG), which are susceptible to motion artifacts and are performed using large apparatuses. Conversely, we expect fNIRS to occupy a unique position among neuroimaging methods: to provide complementary usage in clinical settings, such as bedside situations, for the purposes of diagnosis and treatment [8].

Indeed, fNIRS has been applied in various clinical studies including assessment of the outcome of neurologic rehabilitation for pathological gait [12], monitoring of ischemia [13], monitoring of language dominance before neurosurgery [14], identification of epileptic focus [15, 16], making a diagnosis of various neurological and psychiatric diseases [8, 17], and so on. Furthermore, in Japan, the first clinical applications of fNIRS in neurosurgery, assessment of hemispheric dominance for language function [14], detection of epileptic focus [15], and aid for differential diagnosis of depressive symptoms, have been included under National Health Insurance coverage. There are, indeed, great expectations for the application of fNIRS in various clinical situations, such as the exploration of objective diagnoses for developmental disorders and dementia as well as treatment assessment of medication intervention and rehabilitation. Among these, one of the most promising clinical applications of fNIRS, for which its convenience and robustness would be highly appreciated, is the functional monitoring of ADHD children, who have difficulty performing active cognitive tasks in the enclosed environments of other imaging modalities such as fMRI, PECT, PET, and MEG. A growing body of fNIRS studies has started to investigate the cortical hemodynamics of ADHD patients [18–23].

Attention deficit hyperactivity disorder (ADHD) is one of the most common psychiatric disorders in children. It affects between 3 and 7% of early elementary school children with typical behavioral symptoms of inattention, impulsivity, and hyperactivity [24, 25]. While ADHD is often diagnosed between the ages of 4 and 6 [26], ADHD symptoms are not specific to childhood, and 75–85% of patients are estimated to continue experiencing symptoms through adolescence and adulthood [27]. Consequently, 4–5% of adults have recently been reported to have ADHD [28]. Therefore, early identification and appropriate treatment are considered important in order to increase the quality of life of ADHD patients [29]. Today, the diagnosis of ADHD depends mainly on interview-based evaluation of the degrees of the phenotypes according to diagnostic criteria listed in the DSM-5 as observed by a patient's parents or teachers (http://www.dsm5.org). However, interview-based assessments often entail subjective evaluations by parents and teachers, which present the risk of under or overestimations of ADHD symptoms [30, 31].

ADHD clinical guidelines provide recommended medication treatment, behavioral therapy, and community therapy for ADHD children [32–34]. Furthermore, an American Academy

http://dx.doi.org/10.5772/intechopen.71835

of Pediatrics (AAP) and MTA study revealed that medication treatment was superior to behavioral therapy for school-aged children over 6 years old [35]. According to copious evidence accumulated over several decades, one of the most commonly recommended treatments has been the administration of psychostimulants and non-psychostimulants, such as methylphenidate (MPH) and atomoxetine (ATX) to improve ADHD symptoms [36]. An objective biomarker of the pharmacological effects is urgently required because current treatment evaluation of ADHD depends on evaluation of the degrees of the symptoms listed in the diagnostic criteria. Interview-based measurements need to be rated by parents or teachers of the children, and thus often tend to entail subjective evaluation. Because of the technical limitations of relying on interview-based clinical observation of ADHD patients, the identification of a biological marker is needed to help facilitate objective assessments of pharmacological responses [37–39].

This led us to postulate that fNIRS would be effective in monitoring the effects of the ADHD medications MPH and ATX, especially in younger children who are difficult to assess using other neuroimaging modalities. The lack of evidence associating a neuropharmacological mechanism to therapeutic improvement is tantamount to a missed opportunity for appreciating how MPH and ATX work in the central nervous system, and such understanding is a vital step toward developing an objective, evidence-based neuropharmacological treatment for ADHD children. Thus, we performed an fNIRS study in order to assess acute neuropharmacological effects of MPH and ATX on the inhibitory functions of ADHD children.

We selected a go/no-go task as the experimental task. Go/no-go task has emerged as a principal paradigm for involving the multidimensional construct of response inhibition that refers to the ability to suddenly and completely stop a planned course of action. It is an essential executive function required in daily life, and impaired response inhibition is a strong candidate for a biomarker for ADHD [40] Former fMRI studies successfully visualized decreased hemodynamic responses with ADHD using motor response inhibition tasks including go/no-go, stop signal, and Stroop tasks [41–45]. Among these tasks, go/no-go task performance matures at approximately 12 years [46], followed by stop signal task at 13–17 years, and lastly, Stroop task at around 17–19 years of age [47, 48]. Therefore, a go/no-go task would be the primary choice for a study of school-aged children. fNIRS studies that presented right VLPFC activation during go/no-go tasks have been replicated [9]. Furthermore, structural neuroimaging studies of ADHD have fairly consistently indicated gray matter density reductions in the striatum and right IFG [49].

Therefore, in two consecutive studies making the most of fNIRS's merits, we have explored the neural substrate of inhibitory controls in school-aged ADHD children for the detection of a clinically-oriented biomarker for ADHD diagnosis and evaluation for ADHD medications. In Study 1, we explored differential neural substrates for ADHD and healthy control children during go/no-go task in group analyses using fNIRS measurement. In Study 2, we explored a method of individual differentiation between ADHD and healthy control children using multichannel fNIRS, emphasizing how the spatial distribution and amplitude of hemodynamic response associated with go/no-go task execution can be utilized.

2. Study1: differential neural substrates for ADHD and healthy control children during go/no-go task in group analyses, using fNIRS measurement

Our initial effort [50] examined whether fNIRS-based monitoring for neuropharmacological effects could be visualized in actual clinical situations. To do so, we demonstrated that fNIRS could detect the cortical hemodynamic responses of ADHD children (7–14 years old) performing a go/no-go task before and 1.5 h after MPH administration, allowing the observation of the acute effect of MPH as a significant increase of hemodynamic (oxy-Hb) response in the right prefrontal cortex. As the monitoring takes about 6 minutes, we further demonstrated that the entire protocol can be implemented within a single-day hospital visit.

However, since that study was optimized for assessing the feasibility of fNIRS monitoring as an actual clinical tool that allows the pre- and post-medication comparison to be performed in a single-day hospital visit, a neuro-pharmacological assessment of the effects of ADHD medications has yet to be performed. Experimental designs should be optimized in a neuropharmacological assessment, including a randomized, double-blind design with comparison to healthy control subjects.

Thus, for the present study, to explore the neuropharmacological assessment of ADHD medications, we enrolled ADHD children and age- and sex-matched healthy control subjects, and examined the neuropharmacological effects of ADHD medications on inhibition control, utilizing a within-subject, double-blind, placebo-controlled design. Additionally, we desire to validate the feasibility of introducing fNIRS-based diagnosis of the effects of ADHD medications, MPH and ATX, for use with ADHD children as young as 6 years old, the earliest age at which the FDA recommends starting MPH and ATX administration. **Figure 1** describes the experimental protocol. We examined the effects of MPH (OROS-methylphenidate commercially available as Concerta) and ATX (Strattera, Eli Lilly and Co., Indianapolis, IN, USA) in a randomized, double-blind, placebo-controlled, crossover study during a go/no-go task. All ADHD patients were pre-medicated with MPH (n = 16) or ATX (n = 16) as part of their regular medication regimen. We performed fNIRS measurements of ADHD subjects twice (the times of day for both measurements were scheduled to be as close as possible), at least 2 days apart, but within 30 days. Control subjects underwent a single, non-medicated session. On each examination procedure day, ADHD subjects underwent two sessions, one before drug (MPH/ATX or placebo) administration, and the other 1.5 h after drug administration. Before each pre-administration session, a washout period of 2–3 days was undertaken by all ADHD subjects. Each session involved 6 each of go (baseline) and go/no-go (target) blocks, which were alternated. Each block lasted 24 s and was preceded by trial instructions displayed on a PC monitor for 3 s, giving an overall block-set time of 54 s and a total session time of about 5.5–6.0 min. In the go blocks, we presented subjects with random sequences of two animal pictures and asked them to press a button for both pictures as quickly as possible. In the go/no-go blocks, we presented subjects with a no-go picture 50% of the time, thus requiring subjects to respond to half the trials (go trials) and inhibit their response to the other half (no-go trials). After ADHD subjects performed the first session, either MPH/ATX or a placebo was administered orally. We generated stimuli and collected responses using E-Prime 2.0

http://dx.doi.org/10.5772/intechopen.71835

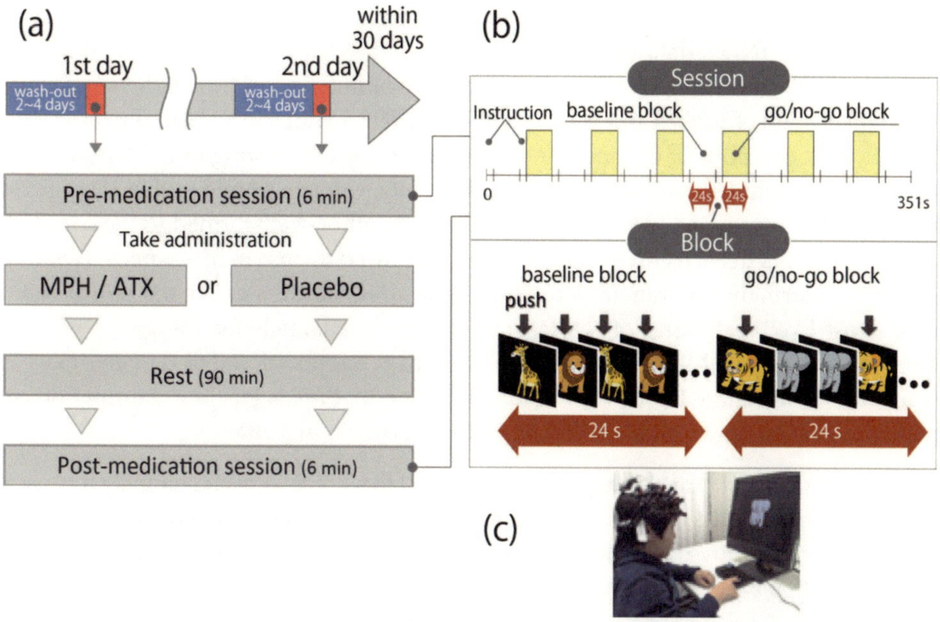

Figure 1. Experimental procedure to detect the differential neural activation pattern for ADHD and healthy control children during go/no-go task in group analyses, using fNIRS measurement. (a) A schematic showing the flow of pre- and post-medication administration sessions for ADHD subjects. (b and c) fNIRS measurements. Brain activity was measured using fNIRS, while ADHD and healthy control subjects performed the go/no-go task.

(Psychology Software Tools). Stimuli were presented to the subject on a 17″ desktop computer screen. The distance between the subject's eyes and the screen was about 50 cm.

We used the multichannel fNIRS system ETG-4000 (Hitachi Medical Corporation, Kashiwa, Japan), which utilizes two wavelengths of near-infrared light (695 and 830 nm). We analyzed the optical data based on the modified Beer-Lambert Law [51] as previously described [52]. This method enabled us to calculate signals reflecting oxygenated hemoglobin (oxy-Hb), deoxygenated hemoglobin (deoxy-Hb), and total hemoglobin (total-Hb) signal changes, obtained in units of millimolar·millimeter (mM·mm) [52]. In order to perform statistical analyses, we treated the oxy-Hb signal as the primary outcome of hemodynamic responses because of its higher sensitivity to changes in cerebral blood flow compared with deoxy-Hb and total-Hb signals [53–55], its higher signal-to-noise ratio [53], and its higher retest reliability [56]. We used two sets of 3x5 multichannel probe holders, which resulted in 22 channels (CH) per set. Each probe holder consisted of eight illuminating and seven detecting probes arranged alternately at an inter-probe distance of 3 cm to cover the lateral prefrontal cortices and inferior parietal lobe, referring to previous studies [9, 57–60]. The midpoint of a pair of illuminating and detecting probes was defined as a channel location. The bilateral probe holders were attached in the following manner: (1) their upper anterior corners, where we connected the right and left probe holders by a belt, were symmetrically placed across the sagittal midline, (2) the lower anterior corners of the probe holder were placed over the supraorbital prominence, and (3) the lower edges of the probe holders were attached at the upper part of the auricles. Virtual registration was adopted for spatial profiling of fNIRS data [61, 62] to register fNIRS data to MNI standard brain space [63]. This method enables us to place a virtual probe holder on the scalp based on a simulation of the holder's deformation and the registration of probes and channels onto reference brains in an MRI database [64, 65]. Specifically, the positions of channels and reference points, consisting of the Nz (nasion), Cz (midline central), and left and right preauricular points, were measured with a 3D-digitizer in real-world (RW) space. The RW reference points were affine-transformed to the corresponding reference points in each entry in reference to the MRI database in MNI space. We adopted the same transformation parameters to obtain the MNI coordinates for the fNIRS channels and the most likely estimates of the locations of given channels for the group of subjects together with the spatial variability associated with the estimation [66]. Finally, macroanatomical labels were estimated using a Matlab function that reads labeling information coded in macroanatomical brain atlases, LBPA40 [67] and Brodmann's atlas [68].

Individual timeline data for the oxy-Hb and deoxy-Hb signals of each channel were preprocessed with a first-degree polynomial fitting and high-pass filter using cut-off frequencies of 0.01 Hz in order to remove baseline drift, and a 0.8 Hz low-pass filter to remove heartbeat pulsations. In fNIRS measurements, note that the Hb signals analyzed do not directly represent cortical Hb concentration changes, but contain an unknown optical path length that cannot be measured. Direct comparison of Hb signals among different channels and regions should be avoided as optical path length is known to vary among cortical regions [69]. Hence, statistical analyses were performed in a channel-wise manner. We computed channel-wise and subject-wise contrasts by calculating the inter-trial mean of differences in Hb signals between peak (4–24 s after go/no-go block onset) and baseline (14–24 s after go block onset) periods from the preprocessed time series data. We visually inspected the movements of the subjects and removed the blocks with sudden, obvious, discontinuous noise for the six go/no-go blocks. We subjected the resulting contrasts to second-level, random-effects group analyses.

Figure 2 describes the experimental results. The oxy-Hb signals were statistically analyzed in a channel-wise manner. Specifically, for healthy control subjects, who were examined only once, a target (no-go block session) vs. baseline (go block session) contrast was generated (**Figure 2(a)**). For ADHD subjects, we generated the following contrasts: (1) pre-medication contrasts: target vs. baseline contrasts for pre-medication conditions (either placebo or MPH/ATX administration) for the first day exclusively (**Figure 2(b)**), (2) post-medication contrasts: the respective target vs. baseline contrasts for post-placebo and post-MPH/ATX conditions (**Figure 2(c, d)**), and (3) inter-medication contrasts: differences between MPH/ATX$^{post\text{–}pre}$ and placebo$^{post\text{–}pre}$ contrasts (**Figure 2(c, d)**). Cortical activation patterns of healthy control subjects (a) and of ADHD subjects (b–d) are shown as t-maps of oxy-Hb signal, with significant *t*-values (one-sample *t*-test, $p < 0.05$) being shown according to the color bar.

Firstly, to screen the channels involved in go/no-go tasks in healthy control subjects, paired t-tests (two-tails) were performed on target vs. baseline contrasts. The statistical threshold was set at 0.05 with Bonferroni correction for family-wise errors. We found significant oxy-Hb increase in the right CH 10 (mean 0.075, SD 0.074, $p < 0.05$, Bonferroni-corrected, Cohen's $d = 1.009$; (**Figure 2(a)**). CH 10 was located in the border region between the right MFG and IFG (MNI

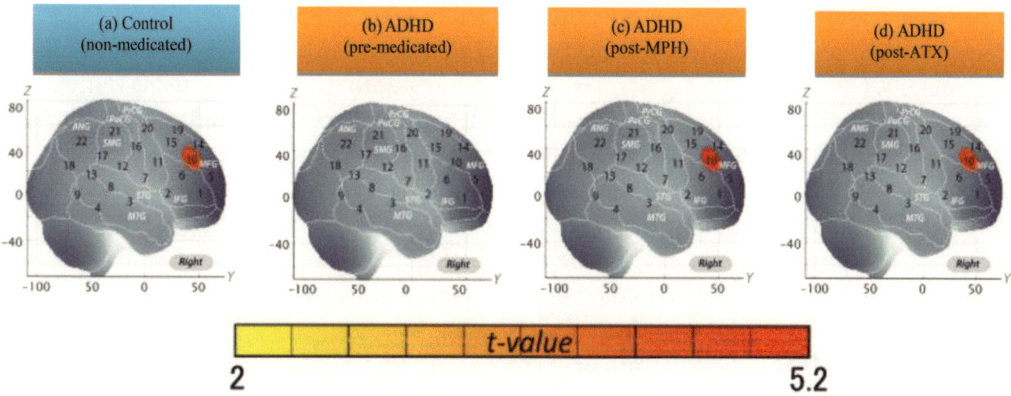

Figure 2. Differences of neuroactivation patterns between ADHD and healthy control during go/no-go task. The channel location of oxy-Hb signals for the right CH 10. (a) Healthy control (b) pre-medicated ADHD (c) post-MPH administration and (d) post-ATX administration.

coordinates *x*, *y*, *z* (SD): 46, 43, 30 (14), MFG 78%, IFG 22% with reference to macroanatomical brain atlases [67, 68]). Therefore, we set the right CH 10 as a region-of-interest (ROI) for the rest of the study. In ADHD conditions, we found that no channels were activated in the pre-medication and post-placebo conditions (**Figure 2(b)**). On the other hand, the right CH 10 exhibited significant oxy-Hb increase in the post-MPH (mean 0.077, SD 0.060, $p < 0.05$, Cohen's $d = 1.283$; (**Figure 2(c)**) and post-ATX (mean 0.074, SD 0.063, $p < 0.05$, Cohen's $d = 1.165$; (**Figure 2(d)**) conditions. Finally, the effects of medications were investigated in the inter-medication contrast: we found the right CH 10 to be significantly different between medication and placebo conditions, MPH (paired *t*-test, $p < 0.05$, Cohen's $d = 0.952$) and ATX (paired *t*-test, $p < 0.05$, Cohen's $d = 0.663$). These results demonstrate that MPH and ATX, but not the placebo, induced an oxy-Hb signal increase during the go/no-go task.

3. Study 1: Discussion

Previous fMRI measurements for healthy control subjects have provided preliminary evidence for the neural correlates of go/no-go tasks [70], including the bilateral IFG, MFG and SFG (superior frontal gyrus), supplementary motor area, anterior cingulate gyrus, inferior parietal and temporal lobes, caudate nucleus, and cerebellum [60]. In addition, recent fMRI [41–45] and fNIRS [71, 72] studies on acute medication effects on ADHD have also shown that bilateral IFG and MFG were robustly normalized after ADHD medications. Taken together, the specificity of the implicated brain regions, such as MFG and IFG, in healthy subjects, as well as functional and structural changes to those regions in ADHD patients, suggests that response inhibition is a good neuro-functional biomarker candidate for ADHD [73].

Our current study found activation in the right MFG and IFG (BA9, 46, 45) during the go/no-go task period in the healthy control subjects, but not in the pre-medicated ADHD subjects. These results suggest that ADHD produces impairment of right prefrontal function associated with go/no-go task performance. The administration of MPH and ATX led to a degree of right prefrontal activation in ADHD children comparable to that of the healthy control subjects, but the placebo did not. These results suggest that as observed using fNIRS, normalized right IFG/MFG activation associated with inhibition control would serve as a robust neurobiological marker for evaluating both MPH and ATX effects. In summary, we explored the feasibility of introducing fNIRS-based neuropharmacological assessment of the effects of MPH/ATX administration to ADHD children, and concluded that the right IFG and MFG activation could serve as robust objective neurobiological markers to visualize the effects of MPH/ATX on ADHD children based on the following observations.

4. Study 2 individual differentiation between ADHD and healthy control children using multichannel fNIRS, emphasizing how spatial distribution and amplitude of hemodynamic response associated with go/no-go task execution can be utilized

The purpose of Study 2 was to explore the possibility of fNIRS-based single-subject diagnosis with various technical approaches. The exploration of fNIRS-based individual classification methodology has been attracting increasing research interest with extremely promising results pertaining to its use for the clinical diagnosis of psychiatric and neurodevelopmental disorders. Recently, a multi-site large-scale fNIRS study involving over 600 adult subjects suffering from bipolar disorder, depressive disorder, and schizophrenia demonstrated high classification accuracy using disorder-specified hemodynamic response patterns: sensitivity of differentiation from healthy control subjects was 76.9% for bipolar disorder, 74.6% for major depressive disorder, and 90.0% for schizophrenia [74]. Furthermore, in a different study enrolling nine boys with medicated ADHD and eight boys with autism spectrum disorder (ASD), use of a support vector machine on hemodynamic response data during a task involving viewing the subject's mother's face allowed the discrimination of the two populations with an 84% accuracy of classification [75].

In our previous session, described above, we introduced fNIRS-based monitoring of the neuropharmacological effects of ADHD medications. Furthermore, with group analyses, we successfully visualized differential neural substrates for ADHD and healthy control children for inhibitory control. The inhibition task recruited the right IFG/MFG, and activation was significantly high during the go/no-go task (Cohen's *d*: 1.009). Those results led us to postulate that right IFG/MFG activations for a go/no-go task, as observed using fNIRS, might be used as an objective neuro-functional biomarker to differentiate school-aged ADHD children and healthy controls at the individual level. Consequently, our next challenge was to explore the inhibition-related dysfunction in ADHD children at an individual level.

We explored a method for individual classification between ADHD and healthy control subjects using fNIRS, emphasizing how spatial distribution and amplitude of the hemodynamic response associated with go/no-go task execution can be utilized. To do this, we needed to identify the cut-off amplitude of cortical activation of each ROI mentioned above in order to differentiate ADHD children from healthy control children. We focused on individual oxy-Hb signal change during target (go/no-go) sessions at multichannel locations for the right MFG and IFG, where a go/no-go-task-related activation in control subjects was conspicuously large at a single-channel location in group analyses from our previous studies [76–78]. In order to identify a robust classification parameter, we adopted the right MFG and IFG as ROIs (call optimized ROIs). Then, making the best use of multichannel analysis, we adapted well-formed formulae to identify the constituent CHs of the optimized ROIs, and assessed whether a specific logic could improve the efficacy of classification.

First, we screened for any fNIRS channels involved in the go/no-go task for control and ADHD subjects at the group level (**Figure 4**). We found significant oxy-Hb increase in three CHs in the right (R) hemisphere, including R CH 5 (mean 0.057, SD 0.077, $p < 0.05$, Bonferroni-corrected, Cohen's $d = 0.741$), R CH 6 (mean 0.046, SD 0.060, $p < 0.05$, Bonferroni-corrected, Cohen's $d = 0.755$), and R CH 10 (mean 0.068, SD 0.065, $p < 0.05$, Bonferroni-corrected, Cohen's $d = 1.046$) in control subjects. Conversely, ADHD conditions showed no significant oxy-Hb increase in the measured cortical areas. Thus, we adopted CHs 5, 6, and 10 as statistically specific ROIs to represent the channels activated for go/no-go task execution in healthy control subjects. We performed independent two-sample *t*-tests (two-tails) on these contrasts with a statistical threshold of $p < 0.05$.

Second, we assessed the group difference in oxy-Hb signals among the ROIs (**Figure 3**). The comparison between ADHD and healthy control subjects revealed significant activation of oxy-Hb signal in the right CHs 6 and 10 in the control subjects than in ADHD subjects at the group level (independent two-sample *t*-test; R CH 6, $p < 0.05$ Bonferroni-corrected, Cohen's $d = 0.964$; R CH 10, $p < 0.05$ Bonferroni-corrected, Cohen's $d = 0.699$). The right CHs 6 and 10 were located in the border region between the right MFG and IFG (R CH 6, MNI coordinates *x*, *y*, *z* (SD): 59, 28, 19 (25), MFG 18%, IFG 52%; R CH 10, MNI coordinates *x*, *y*, *z* (SD): 48, 37, 34 (27), MFG 63%, IFG 31%) in reference to a macroanatomical brain atlas [68].

We applied CHs 6 and 10 as statistically robust ROIs to represent the most significant activation in healthy control compared with ADHD subjects during go/no-go task execution. In order to

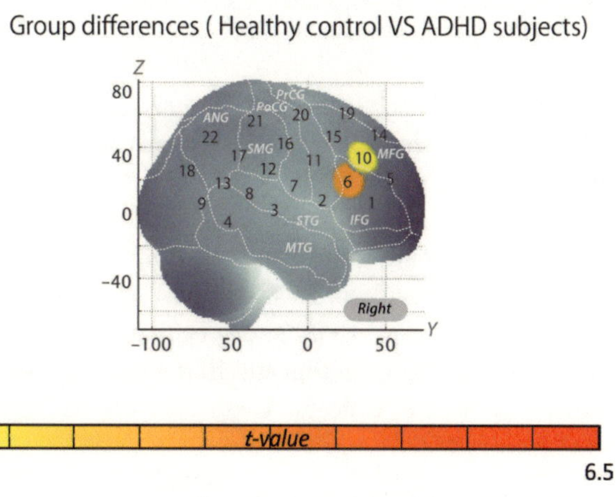

Figure 3. Cortical activation patterns for group-level comparison between the ADHD and healthy control groups during a go/no-go task. t-Maps of oxy-Hb signals are displayed, with significant *t*-values (paired *t*-test, Bonferroni-corrected) shown according to the color bar.

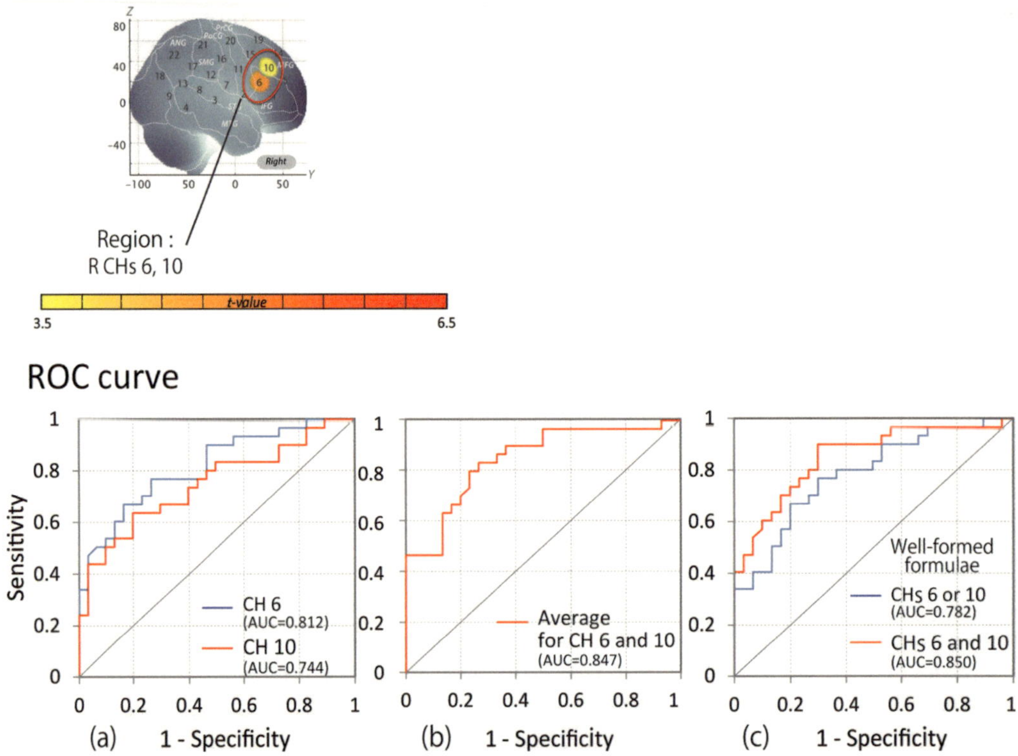

Figure 4. In order to predict ADHD diagnosis using channel-wised hemodynamic changes, we applied CHs 6 and 10 as statistically robust ROIs to represent the most significant activation in healthy control compared with ADHD subjects during go/no-go task execution. We explored setting a cut-off value for individual fNIRS-based oxy-Hb signal patterns: (a) CHs 6 and 10, respectively, (b) average oxy-Hb signal contrasts for the right CHs 6 and 10, (c) optimized values using well-formed formulae. For each cut-off value, sensitivity and 1-specificity to create a receiver operating characteristic (ROC) were plotted. Subsequently, the area under the resultant ROC curve (AUC) was calculated. Finally, the best cut-off value was identified as that with the highest sensitivity and specificity, which is the point nearest to the top left corner of the curve.

classify ADHD and healthy control children with higher accuracy, we explored setting a cut-off value for individual fNIRS-based oxy-Hb signal patterns. We set the initial cut-off value for the oxy-Hb signal at 0 mM·mm. From this start point, the cut-off value was incremented or diminished until specificity or sensitivity reached 0 or 1. For each cut-off value, we plotted sensitivity and 1-specificity to create a receiver operating characteristic (ROC). In addition, we calculated the area under the resultant ROC curve (AUC). Then the best cut-off value was identified as that with the highest sensitivity and specificity, which is the point nearest to the top left corner of the curve (**Figure 4**). In this and in the previous study, the PASW Statistics (version 18 for Windows) (SPSS Inc., Chicago, USA) software package was used for statistical analyses.

First, we examined each channel (CH 6 and 10) component. For CH 6, the AUC value was 81.20%. At the optimal cut-off value of 0.0000 mM·mm, differentiation between ADHD and healthy control subjects was achieved with a sensitivity of 66.7% and a specificity of

83.3% (**Figure 4(a)**). For CH 10, the AUC value was 74.4%. At the optimal cut-off value of 0.0320 mM·mm, differentiation between ADHD and healthy control subjects was achieved with a sensitivity of 63.3% and a specificity of 80.0% (**Figure 4(a)**). Second, the averages of the integral values for CHs 6 and 10 for 30 individual ADHD and healthy control subjects were calculated (**Figure 4(b)**). The resulting AUC value was 84.7%. At the optimal cut-off value of 0.0374 mM·mm, differentiation between ADHD and healthy control subjects was achieved with a sensitivity of 83.3% and a specificity of 73.3% (**Figure 4(a)**).

Third, for further optimization, we adapted well-formed formulae for CHs 6 and 10 in the most optimized ROI. With "AND" logic, a subject was classified as normal (not ADHD), when the subject's oxy-Hb signals for CHs 6 "AND" 10 were above a given threshold. When "OR" logic was applied, a subject was classified as normal (not ADHD), when the subject's oxy-Hb signal for CH 6 "OR" 10 was above a given threshold. For each classification using well-formed formulae, ROC analysis was performed as described above. We adapted well-formed formulae for CHs 6 and 10 to better classify ADHD and healthy control subjects. When "OR" logic was adopted, the area under the AUC was 78.2%. At the optimal cut-off value of 0.0650 mM·mm, differentiation between ADHD and healthy control subjects was achieved with a sensitivity of 76.7% and a specificity of 70.0% (**Figure 4**). Finally, when "AND" logic was adopted, the AUC value was 85.0%, which was the highest percentage among all classifications. At the optimal cut-off value of 0.0111 mM·mm, differentiation between ADHD and healthy control subjects was achieved with a sensitivity of 90.0% and a specificity of 70.0% (**Figure 4**).

5. Study 2: Discussion

Optimized ROIs in the right IFG and MFG to differentiate ADHD children from healthy control children were successfully identified through individual assessment of channel-wise oxy-Hb signal changes using fNIRS; adaptation of well-formed formulae to two CHs to form optimized ROIs achieved 90% sensitivity for diagnostic predictions at the individual level. Thus, we suggest the high possibility that this novel fNIRS-based measurement may serve as an efficient diagnostic method to enable differentiation between ADHD and healthy children at an individual level. Previous neuroimaging studies have reported on methods for diagnostic classification of ADHD and healthy control subjects at the individual level that adopt multifactorial methods (e.g., neuroanatomical pattern classification) to structural MRI data [43, 79] and to fMRI data [37, 80–84]. However, our protocol requires only a single variable (the simple "integral value" of fNIRS signals for only two ROIs) and produces high classification rates (sensitivity: 90%). Our classification rates were equivalent to those reported for previous MRI and fMRI studies using multivariate statistical methods, which ranged from 67 to 93% for ADHD groups compared with healthy control children.

Recently, a considerable number of studies have introduced neural correlates for go/no-go tasks, including the right IFG and MFG [60]. Furthermore, a recent activation likelihood estimation (ALE) meta-analysis of go/no-go tasks [85] revealed a mainly right-lateralized network associated with response inhibition, including the right MFG and IFG (BA46/44) [70].

The right IFG and MFG have been implicated in processes of response selection, stimulus recognition, and maintenance and manipulation of stimulus-response associations, including selecting not to respond, all of which are critical in the performance of go/no-go tasks.

From a genetic perspective, the catechol-O-methyltransferase (COMT) gene [86], the dopamine active transporter 1 gene (DAT1, also known as SLC6A3), and the dopamine receptor D4 (DRD4) gene [39] are deeply associated with the pathophysiology of ADHD. These genes are thought to be involved in the monoamine system, and their dysfunction in the prefrontal cortex, including the IFG and MFG, is considered to be the core pathomechanism of ADHD.

6. Limitations Study 1 & 2

As discussed above, the current study has demonstrated that our fNIRS-based experimental method of using inhibition-elicited cerebral functional to differentiate between ADHD and healthy control children allows the observation of a distinct biological marker in clinical situations. However, before establishing its utility in clinical practice, several issues need to be addressed.

First, the scope of the current study does not necessarily extend to screening for ADHD with comorbidity. Therefore, our next step is to explore the disorder-specificity of fNIRS-based individual classification relative to other developmental and psychiatric disorders, such as autism spectrum disorder, oppositional defiant disorder, conduct disorder, depression, and anxiety.

Second, although most ADHD subjects had temporally stopped medication (MPH or ATX) for more than 48 hours before fNIRS examination, the condition of the ADHD subjects in this study may not precisely reflect immune brain activation. Several other neuroimaging studies examining medication-naïve ADHD patients have been reported in a recent meta-analysis [87]. Brain function can be changed with long-term MPH and ATX administration; the recent meta-analysis of human studies using fMRI suggested that long-term MPH treatment is associated with more normal activation in the right DLPFC. Therefore, we need to explore medication-naïve ADHD patients as our next step.

Author details

Yukifumi Monden[1,2,3]*, Masako Nagashima[1], Haruka Dan[2], Takahiro Ikeda[1], Yasushi Kyutoku[2], Takanori Yamagata[1] and Ippeita Dan[2]

*Address all correspondence to: mon4441977319@jichi.ac.jp

1 Department of Pediatrics, Jichi Medical University, Tochigi, Japan

2 Applied Cognitive Neuroscience Laboratory, Chuo University, Tokyo, Japan

3 Department of Pediatrics, International University of Health and Welfare, Tochigi, Japan

References

[1] Obrig H, Villringer A. Beyond the visible-imaging the human brain with light. Journal of Cerebral Blood Flow & Metabolism. 2003;**23**:1-18. DOI: 10.1097/01.WCB.0000043472.45775.29

[2] Strangman G, Boas DA, Sutton JP. Non-invasive neuroimaging using near-infrared light. Biological Psychiatry. 2002;**52**:679-693

[3] Ferrari M, Quaresima V. A brief review on the history of human functional near-infrared spectroscopy (fNIRS) development and fields of application. NeuroImage. 2012;**63**: 921-935. DOI: 10.1016/j.neuroimage.2012.03.049

[4] Minagawa-Kawai Y, Mori K, Hebden JC, et al. Optical imaging of infants' neurocognitive development: Recent advances and perspectives. Developmental Neurobiology. 2008;**68**:712-728. DOI: 10.1002/dneu.20618

[5] Lloyd-Fox S, Blasi SA, Elwell CE. Illuminating the developing brain: The past, present and future of functional near infrared spectroscopy. Neuroscience and Biobehavioral Reviews. 2010;**34**:269-284. DOI: 10.1016/j.neubiorev.2009.07.008

[6] Okamoto M, Dan H, Shimizu K, et al. Multimodal assessment of cortical activation during apple peeling by NIRS and fMRI. NeuroImage. 2004;**21**:1275-1288. DOI: 10.1016/j.neuroimage.2003.12.003

[7] Hock C, Villringer K, Muller-Sphan F, et al. Decrease in parietal cerebral hemoglobin oxygenation during performance of a verbal fluency task in patients with Alzheimer's disease monitored by means of near-infrared spectroscopy (NIRS) – correlation with simultaneous rCBF-PET measurements. Brain Research. 1997;**755**:293-303

[8] Suto T, Fukuda M, Ito M, et al. Multichannel near-infrared spectroscopy in depression and schizophrenia: Cognitive brain activation study. Biological Psychiatry. 2004;**55**: 501-511. DOI: 10.1016/j.biopsych.2003.09.008

[9] Herrmann MJ, Plichta MM, Ehlis AC, et al. Optical topography during a Go-NoGo task assessed with multi-channel near-infrared spectroscopy. Behavioural Brain Research. 2005;**160**:135-140. DOI: 10.1016/j.bbr.2004.11.032

[10] Okamoto M, Matsunami M, Dan H, et al. Prefrontal activity during taste encoding: An fNIRS study. NeuroImage. 2006;**31**:796-806. DOI: 10.1016/j.neuroimage.2005.12.021

[11] Moriai-Izawa A. Multichannel fNIRS assessment of overt and covert confrontation naming. Brain and Language. 2012;**121**:185-193

[12] Miyai I, Dan H, Dan I, et al. Cortical mapping of gait in humans: A near-infrared spectroscopic topography study. NeuroImage. 2001;**14**:1186-1192. DOI: 10.1016/j.bandl.2012.02.001

[13] Murata Y, Sakatani K, Katayama Y, et al. Increase in focal concentration of deoxyhaemoglobin during neuronal activity in cerebral ischaemic patients. Journal of Neurology, Neurosurgery, and Psychiatry. 2002;**73**:182-184

[14] Watanabe E, Maki A, Kawaguchi F, et al. Noninvasive cerebral blood volume measurement during seizures using multichannel near infrared spectroscopic topography. Journal of Biomedical Optics. 2000;**5**:287-290. DOI: 10.1117/1.429998

[15] Watanabe E, Nagahori Y, Mayanagi Y, Focus Y. Diagnosis of epilepsy using near-infrared spectroscopy. Epilepsia. 2002;**43**:50-55

[16] Nguyen DK, Tremblay J, Pouliot P, et al. Noninvasive continuous functional near-infrared spectroscopy combined with electroencephalography recording of frontal lobe seizures. Epilepsia. 2012;**54**:331-340. DOI: 10.1111/epi.12011

[17] Hahn T, Marquand AF, Plichta MM, et al. A novel approach to probabilistic biomarker-based classification using functional near-infrared spectroscopy. Human Brain Mapping. 2012;**34**:1102-1114. DOI: 10.1002/hbm.21497

[18] Weber P, Lutschg J, Fahnenstich H, Cerebral H. Hemodynamic changes in response to an executive function task in children with attention-deficit hyperactivity disorder measured by near-infrared spectroscopy. Journal of Developmental and Behavioral Pediatrics. 2005;**26**:105-111

[19] Ehlis AC, Bähne CG, Jacob CP, et al. Reduced lateral prefrontal activation in adult patients with attention-deficit/hyperactivity disorder (ADHD) during a working memory task: A functional near-infrared spectroscopy (fNIRS) study. Journal of Psychiatric Research. 2008;**42**:1060-1067. DOI: 10.1016/j.jpsychires.2007.11.011

[20] Schecklmann M, Ehlis AC, Plichta MM, et al. Diminished prefrontal oxygenation with normal and above-average verbal fluency performance in adult ADHD. Journal of Psychiatric Research. 2008;**43**:98-106. DOI: 10.1016/j.jpsychires.2008.02.005

[21] Schecklmann M, Romanos M, Bretscher F, et al. Prefrontal oxygenation during working memory in ADHD. Journal of Psychiatric Research. 2010;**44**:621-628. DOI: 10.1016/j.jpsychires.2009.11.018

[22] Negoro H, Sawada M, Iida J, et al. Prefrontal dysfunction in attention-deficit/hyperactivity disorder as measured by near-infrared spectroscopy. Child Psychiatry and Human Development. 2010;**41**:193-203. DOI: 10.1007/s10578-009-0160-y

[23] Inoue Y, Sakihara K, Gunji A, et al. Reduced prefrontal hemodynamic response in children with ADHD during the go/no-go task: A NIRS study. Neuroreport. 2011;**23**:55-60. DOI: 10.1097/WNR.0b013e32834e664c.

[24] Dittmann RW, Wehmeier PM, Schacht A, et al. Atomoxetine treatment and ADHD-related difficulties as assessed by adolescent patients, their parents and physicians. Child Adolesc Psychiatry Ment Health. 2009;**3**(1):21. DOI: 10.1186/1753-2000-3-21

[25] Craig F, Margari F, Legrottaglie AR, et al. A review of executive function deficits in autism spectrum disorder and attention-deficit/hyperactivity disorder. Neuropsychiatric Disease and Treatment. 2016;**12**:1191-1202. DOI: 10.2147/NDT.S104620.eCollection 2016

[26] Drechsler R, Brandeis D, Földényi M, et al. The course of neuropsychological functions in children with attention deficit hyperactivity disorder from late childhood to early adolescence. Journal of Child Psychology and Psychiatry. 2005;**46**:824-836

[27] Lahey BB, Applegate B, Waldman ID, et al. The structure of child and adolescent psychopathology: Generating new hypotheses. Journal of Abnormal Psychology. 2004;**113**:358-385

[28] Safren SA, Sprich S, Mimiaga MJ, et al. Cognitive behavioral therapy vs relaxation with educational support for medication-treated adults with ADHD and persistent symptoms: A randomized controlled trial. Journal of the American Medical Association. 2010;**304**:875-880. DOI: 10.1001/jama.2010.1192

[29] Power TJ, Shapiro ES, DuPaul GJ. Preparing psychologists to link systems of care in managing and preventing children's health problems. Journal of Pediatric Psychology. 2003;**28**:147-155

[30] Bruchmuller K, Margraf J, Schneider S. Is ADHD diagnosed in accord with diagnostic criteria? Overdiagnosis and influence of client gender on diagnosis. Journal of Consulting and Clinical Psychology. 2012;**80**:128-138. DOI: 10.1037/a0026582

[31] Batstra L, Hadders-Algra M, Nieweg E, et al. Childhood emotional and behavioral problems: Reducing overdiagnosis without risking undertreatment. Developmental Medicine and Child Neurology. 2012;**54**:492-494. DOI: 10.1111/j.1469-8749.2011.04176.x

[32] Wolraich M, Brown L, Brown RT, et al. ADHD: Clinical practice guideline for the diagnosis, evaluation, and treatment of attention-deficit/hyperactivity disorder in children and adolescents. Pediatrics. 2011;**128**:1007-1022. DOI: 10.1542/peds.2011-2654

[33] Pliszka S. Practice parameter for the assessment and treatment of children and adolescents with attention-deficit/hyperactivity disorder. Journal of the American Academy of Child and Adolescent Psychiatry. 2007;**46**:894-921

[34] Taylor E, Döpfner M, Sergeant J, et al. European clinical guidelines for hyperkinetic disorder – first upgrade. European Child & Adolescent Psychiatry. 2004;**13**:17-30

[35] Hodgkins P, Shaw M, Coghill D, et al. Amfetamine and methylphenidate medications for attention-deficit/hyperactivity disorder: Complementary treatment options. European Child & Adolescent Psychiatry. 2012;**21**(9):477-492. DOI: 10.1007/s00787-012-0286-5

[36] Spencer TJ. ADHD treatment across the life cycle. The Journal of Clinical Psychiatry. 2004;**65**:22-26

[37] Zhu CZ, Zang YF, Cao QJ, et al. Fisher discriminative analysis of resting-state brain function for attention-deficit/hyperactivity disorder. NeuroImage. 2008;**40**:110-120. DOI: 10.1016/j.neuroimage.2007.11.029

[38] Wehmeier PM, Schacht A, Barkley RA. Social and emotional impairment in children and adolescents with ADHD and the impact on quality of life. The Journal of Adolescent Health. 2010;**46**:209-217. DOI: 10.1016/j.jadohealth.2009.09.009

[39] Leitner Y. The co-occurrence of autism and attention deficit hyperactivity disorder in children – What do we know? Frontiers in Human Neuroscience. 2014;**8**:268. DOI: 10.3389/fnhum.2014.00268. eCollection 2014

[40] Barkley RA. Behavioral inhibition, sustained attention, and executive functions: Constructing a unifying theory of ADHD. Psychological Bulletin. 1997;**121**:65-94

[41] Dillo W, Göke A, Prox-Vagedes V, et al. Neuronal correlates of ADHD in adults with evidence for compensation strategies – A functional MRI study with a go/no-go paradigm. German Medical Science. 2010;**8**:9. DOI: 10.3205/000098

[42] Bush G, Frazier JA, Rauch SL, et al. Anterior cingulate cortex dysfunction in attention-deficit/hyperactivity disorder revealed by fMRI and the counting Stroop. Biological Psychiatry. 1999;**45**:1542-1552

[43] Durston S, Tottenham NT, Thomas KM, et al. Differential patterns of striatal activation in young children with and without ADHD. Biological Psychiatry. 2003;**53**:871-878

[44] Vaidya CJ, Austin G, Kirkorian G, et al. Selective effects of methylphenidate in attention deficit hyperactivity disorder: A functional magnetic resonance study. Proceedings of the National Academy of Sciences of the United States of America. 1998;**95**:14494-14499

[45] Rubia K, Overmeyer S, Taylor E, et al. Hypofrontality in attention deficit hyperactivity disorder during higher-order motor control: A study with functional MRI. The American Journal of Psychiatry. 1999;**156**(6):891

[46] Levin HS et al. Developmental changes in performance on tests of purported frontal lobe functioning. Developmental Neuropsychology. 1991;**7**:377-395

[47] Comalli PE, Wapner S Jr, Werner H. Interference effects of Stroop color-word test in childhood, adulthood, and aging. The Journal of Genetic Psychology. 1962;**100**:47-53

[48] Williams BR, Ponesse JS, Schachar RJ, et al. Development of inhibitory control across the life span. Developmental Psychology. 1999;**35**(1):205-213

[49] Durston S, Hulshoff Pol HE, Schnack HG, et al. Magnetic resonance imaging of boys with attention-deficit/hyperactivity disorder and their unaffected siblings. Journal of the American Academy of Child and Adolescent Psychiatry. 2004;**43**:332-340

[50] Monden Y, Dan H, Nagashima M, et al. Clinically-oriented monitoring of acute effects of methylphenidate on cerebral hemodynamics in ADHD children using fNIRS. Clinical Neurophysiology. 2011;**123**:1147-1157. DOI: 10.1016/j.clinph.2011.10.006.

[51] Cope M, Delpy DT, Reynolds EO, et al. Methods of quantitating cerebral near infrared spectroscopy data. Adv Exp Med Biol. 1988;**222**:183-189

[52] Maki A, Yamashita Y, Ito Y, Watanabe E, et al. Spatial and temporal analysis of human motor activity using noninvasive NIR topography. Medical Physics. 1995;**22**:1997-2005

[53] Strangman G, Culver JP, Thompson JH, et al. A quantitative comparison of simultaneous BOLD fMRI and NIRS recordings during functional brain activation. NeuroImage. 2002;**17**:719-731

[54] Hoshi Y, Kobayashi N, Tamura M. Interpretation of near-infrared spectroscopy signals: A study with a newly developed perfused rat brain model. Journal of Applied Physiology. 2001;**90**:1657-1662

[55] Hoshi Y. Functional near-infrared optical imaging: Utility and limitations in human brain mapping. Psychophysiology. 2003;**40**:511-520

[56] Plichta M, Herrmann MJ, Baehne CG, et al. Event-related functional near-infrared spectroscopy (fNIRS): Are the measurements reliable? NeuroImage. 2006;**31**:116-124

[57] Garavan H, Ross TJ, Stein EA. Right hemispheric dominance of inhibitory control: An event-related functional MRI study. Proceedings of the National Academy of Sciences of the United States of America. 1999;**96**:8301-8306

[58] Herrmann M, Ehlis AC, Fallgatter A. Bilaterally reduced frontal activation during a verbal fluency task in depressed patients as measured by near-infrared spectroscopy. The Journal of Neuropsychiatry and Clinical Neurosciences. 2004;**16**:170-175

[59] Liddle PF, Kiehl KA, Smith AM. Event-related fMRI study of response inhibition. Human Brain Mapping. 2001;**12**:100-109

[60] Rubia K, Smith AB, Brammer MJ, et al. Right inferior prefrontal cortex mediates response inhibition while mesial prefrontal cortex is responsible for error detection. NeuroImage. 2003;**20**:351-358

[61] Tsuzuki D, Dan I. Spatial registration for functional near-infrared spectroscopy: From channel position on the scalp to cortical location in individual and group analyses. NeuroImage. 2014;**85**:92-103. DOI: 10.1016/j.neuroimage.2013.07.025

[62] Tsuzuki D, Jurcak V, Singh AK, et al. Virtual spatial registration of stand-alone fNIRS data to MNI space. NeuroImage. 2007;**34**:1506-1518

[63] Brett M, Johnsrude LS, Owen AM. The problem of functional localization in the human brain. Nature Reviews Neuroscience. 2002;**3**:243-249

[64] Okamoto M, Dan H, Sakamoto K, et al. Three-dimensional probabilistic anatomical cranio-cerebral correlation via the international 10-20 system oriented for transcranial functional brain mapping. NeuroImage. 2004;**21**:99-111

[65] Okamoto M, Dan I. Automated cortical projection of head-surface locations for transcranial functional brain mapping. NeuroImage. 2005;**26**(1):18-28

[66] Singh AK, Dan I. Exploring the false discovery rate in multichannel NIRS. NeuroImage. 2006;**33**:542-549

[67] Shattuck DW, Mirza M, Adisetiyo V, et al. Construction of a 3D probabilistic atlas of human cortical structures. NeuroImage. 2008;**39**:1064-1080

[68] Rorden C, Brett M. Stereotaxic display of brain lesions. Behavioural Neurology. 2000;**12**:191-200

[69] Katagiri A, Dan I, Tuzuki D, et al. Mapping of optical pathlength of human adult head at multi-wavelengths in near infrared spectroscopy. Adv Exp Med Biol. pp. 205-212. DOI: 10.1007/978-1-4419-1241-1_29, 10.1007/978-1-4419-1241-1_29

[70] Simmonds DJ, Pekar JJ, Mostofsky SH. Meta-analysis of go/no-go tasks demonstrating that fMRI activation associated with response inhibition is task-dependent. Neuropsychologia. 2008;**46**:224-232

[71] Araki A, Ikegami M, Okayama A, et al. Improved prefrontal activity in AD/HD children treated with atomoxetine: A NIRS study. Brain & Development. 2015;**37**:76-87. DOI: 10.1016/j.braindev.2014.03.011

[72] Ishii-Takahashi A, Takizawa R, Nishimura Y, et al. Neuroimaging-aided prediction of the effect of methylphenidate in children with attention-deficit hyperactivity disorder: A randomized controlled trial. Neuropsychopharmacology. 2015;**40**:2676-2685. DOI: 10.1038/npp.2015.154

[73] Aron AR, Poldrack RA. The cognitive neuroscience of response inhibition: Relevance for genetic research in attention-deficit/hyperactivity disorder. Biological Psychiatry. 2005;**57**:1285-1292

[74] Takizawa R, Fukuda M, Kawasaki S, et al. Neuroimaging-aided differential diagnosis of the depressive state. NeuroImage. 2014;**85**:498-507. DOI: 10.1016/j.neuroimage.2013.05.126

[75] Ichikawa H, Kitazono J, Nagata K, et al. Novel method to classify hemodynamic response obtained using multi-channel fNIRS measurements into two groups: Exploring the combinations of channels. Frontiers in Human Neuroscience. 2014;**8**:480. DOI: 10.3389/fnhum.2014.00480.eCollection 2014

[76] Monden Y, Dan H, Nagashima M, et al. Right prefrontal activation as a neuro-functional biomarker for monitoring acute effects of methylphenidate in ADHD children: An fNIRS study. NeuroImage: Clinical. 2012;**1**:131-140. DOI: 10.1016/j.nicl.2012.10.001.eCollection 2012

[77] Monden Y, Dan H, Nagashima M, et al. Clinically-oriented monitoring of acute effects of methylphenidate on cerebral hemodynamics in ADHD children using fNIRS. Clinical Neurophysiology. 2012;**123**:1147-1157. DOI: 10.1016/j.clinph.2011.10.006 Epub Nov 15, 2011

[78] Nagashima M, Monden Y, Dan I, et al. Acute neuropharmacological effects of atomoxetine on inhibitory control in ADHD children: A fNIRS study. NeuroImage: Clinical. 2014;**6**:192-201. DOI: 10.1016/j.nicl.2014.09.001.eCollection 2014

[79] Johnston BA, Mwangi B, Matthews K, et al. Brainstem abnormalities in attention deficit hyperactivity disorder support high accuracy individual diagnostic classification. Human Brain Mapping. 2014;**35**:5179-5189. DOI: 10.1002/hbm.22542 Epub May 13, 2014

[80] Solmaz B. ADHD classification using bag of words approach on network features. In: SPIE Medical Imaging. International Society for Optics and Photonics; 2012

[81] Colby JB. Insights into multimodal imaging classification of ADHD. Frontiers in Systems Neuroscience. 2012;**16**;6:59. DOI: 10.3389/fnsys.2012.00059. eCollection 2012

[82] Dai D, Rudie JD, Brown JA, et al. Classification of ADHD children through multimodal magnetic resonance imaging. Frontiers in Systems Neuroscience. 2012;**6**(3):63. DOI: 10.3389/fnsys.2012.00063. eCollection 2012

[83] Hoekzema E, Carmona S, Ramos-Quiroga JA, et al. An independent components and functional connectivity analysis of resting state fMRI data points to neural network dysregulation in adult ADHD. Hum Brain Mapp. Apr; 2014;**35**:1261-1272. DOI: 10.1002/hbm.22250. Epub 2013 Feb 18

[84] Hart H. Pattern classification of response inhibition in ADHD: Toward the development of neurobiological markers for ADHD. Human Brain Mapping. 2014;**35**:3083-3094

[85] Buchsbaum BR, Greer S, Chang WL, et al. Meta-analysis of neuroimaging studies of the Wisconsin card-sorting task and component processes. Human Brain Mapping. 2005;**25**:35-45

[86] Taurines R, Schwenck C, Westerwald E, et al. ADHD and autism: Differential diagnosis or overlapping traits? A selective review. Attention Deficit and Hyperactivity Disorders. 2012;**4**:115-139. DOI: 10.1007/s12402-012-0086-2

[87] Hart H, Radua J, Mataix-Cols D, Rubia K. Meta-analysis of fMRI studies of timing in attention-deficit hyperactivity disorder (ADHD). Neuroscience and Biobehavioral Reviews. 2012;**36**:2248-2256

Chapter 2

The Role of the Magnetic Resonance Imaging for the Accurate Management of Focal Therapy with High-Intensity Focused Ultrasound for the Localized Prostate Cancer

Sunao Shoji and Akira Miyajima

Additional information is available at the end of the chapter

http://dx.doi.org/10.5772/intechopen.71996

Abstract

The concept of the currently attracted focal therapy is to treat clinical significant cancer with minimal invasion of health-related functions such as urethra, sphincter, neurovascular bundle, and bladder neck. The patients' criteria have been decided with pathologic tumor features characterized according to a combination of cancer core length and Gleason grade with prostate biopsy. Because the area involved in a single treatment using high-intensity focused ultrasound (HIFU) is extremely small, only minor temperature changes are observed outside of the focal zone. HIFU has been considered as an attractive therapeutic modality for the focal treatment of the prostate with the aim of curing the cancer while preserving continence and erectile function. Clinical trials of focal ablation of prostate cancer with HIFU have been reported. In our protocol, magnetic resonance imaging (MRI) has played a major role in the diagnosis of the spatial location of the significant cancer, treatment planning, and the evaluation of the treatment efficacy and recurrence after the treatment. In the chapter in "MR Imaging," we want to present the role of MRI in the accurate management of focal therapy with HIFU for the localized prostate cancer.

Keywords: prostate cancer, focal therapy, magnetic resonance imaging, high-intensity focused ultrasound

1. Introduction

High-intensity focused ultrasound (HIFU) produces ultrasound waves generated by a spherical transducer, delivering ultrasonic energy to pinpoint foci millimeters in diameter [1]. The thermal and mechanical effects of HIFU cause destruction within prostate tissue [2, 3]. Specifically, coagulative degeneration quickly develops and is a primary mechanism for decreasing blood flow [3, 4]. Cavitation, a mechanical effect of HIFU, occurs because of the rapid cycling from compression to refraction by the ultrasound waves and results in the formation of microbubbles in tissue. When these bubbles reach the size of resonance, they collapse and produce high-pressure shock waves, destroying adjacent tissue [5]. Clinically, HIFU energy is delivered in a pulsed mode, and pulses are defined by treatment cycles and energy intensity in watts. Pulse characteristics define the size of the ablation area, including necessary margins to ensure full tumor coverage. The resulting tissue effects are a function of the frequency (wavelength) and intensity (I, in W/cm^2) of the applied energy. Intensity is a function of the excitation (voltage) and duration of the energy pulse. The exact size of the ablated area depends on the type of device used, shape of the piezoceramic working element of the transducer, ultrasound frequency and duration of pulsed energy applied, degree of sonication absorption by the tumor tissue, and focal intensity achieved.

Because the area involved in a single treatment using HIFU is extremely small, only minor temperature changes are observed outside of the focal zone [3], making it an attractive therapeutic modality for focal treatment of the prostate, with the aim of curing the cancer while preserving continence and erectile function. Clinical trials of focal ablation of prostate cancers with HIFU have been reported [6–11]. In the management of the focal therapy, MRI has the role in the localization of the targeted lesion, the evaluation of the treatment effectiveness, and the local recurrence after the treatment.

2. The technology of the HIFU in the treatment of the prostate cancer

After the early studies for the treatment of organ-confined prostate cancer, the Sonablate® device and Ablatherm® device have been further enhanced to include treatment planning capabilities and improved therapeutic technologies.

In the treatment planning, the Sonablate® transrectal HIFU probes use proprietary transducer technology with low-energy ultrasound (4 MHz) for imaging of the prostate and high-energy ablative pulses (site intensity: 1300–2200 W/cm^2) for treatment delivery. For the Ablatherm® device, the transrectal HIFU probes use 7.5 MHz pulses for imaging of the prostate and 3 MHz for the delivery of high-energy ablative pulses (site intensity, 1300–2200 W/cm^2). In recent applications of HIFU, the treatment range was planned using a MRI-TRUS fusion image. Additionally, reconstructed three-dimensional (3D) planning modes have been integrated into the SB 500 V4 and AB integrated devices, facilitating accurate planning of treatment range. Because of the inherent technology of HIFU treatments, there is no need to puncture the prostate during treatment; however, this makes accurate treatment planning essential for successful focal HIFU therapy.

In the treatment, intraoperative images are available during the procedure. The "popcorn" phenomena formed by the cavitations of tissue may act as an indicator of treatment efficacy. The SB500 tissue change monitoring system (TCM) predicts treatment efficacy by calculation of radio frequency signal from an area of interest and classifies it based on a 3-color system; green: insufficient change to cure, yellow: moderate change, and orange: large change. Based

http://dx.doi.org/10.5772/intechopen.71996

on the color indicated on the treated area, intraoperative retreatment for an insufficiently treated zone (green area) would then be performed. A recent development in the field of adaptive treatment planning is the Focal One®. This device has a dynamic focusing transducer made of 16 isocentric rings and allows the user to electronically steer the ultrasound beam and move the focal point of the transducer to a maximum of eight different points (32–67 mm from the transducer).

3. The role of MRI in the management of focal therapy

3.1. The localization of the clinically significant cancer in the prostate with MRI-TRUS fusion image-guided prostate biopsy

Multiparametric MRI (mpMRI) improves the imaging of the clinically significant prostate cancer in the prostate [12, 13], and the information of mpMRI has been used for the precise diagnosis and localization of the clinically significant prostate cancer. MRI-TRUS fusion image-guided biopsy achieved accurate prostate biopsy based on MRI, combining the superior sensitivity of MRI for targeting cancer-suspicious lesions with the practicality and familiarity of TRUS. With the MRI-TRUS fusion devices, the stored MRI and real-time TRUS are superimposed using computer software to enable targeted biopsy of cancer-suspicious lesions [14]. MRI-TRUS fusion biopsy device "BioJet®" was approved by FDA after the evaluation of the accuracy with phantoms. We reported the BioJet® experience of the usefulness of the precise diagnosis of the clinically significant cancer [15]. In the 30 patients from whom whole-mount specimens were taken, we found 43 clinically significant cancers, of which 41 (95%) had been detected by both the targeted and systematic biopsies. The median major diameter of significant cancers in the whole-gland specimens was 12 (range: 5–28) mm; lesions ≤10 mm represented 59% of the significant cancers (n = 24). Of the significant cancers ≤10 mm (n = 24) in whole-mount specimens, 96% (n = 23) were correctly diagnosed by biopsy. Gleason scores and locations of biopsy-proven significant cancers corresponded to histopathological findings for the whole-mount specimens, since the localization of the clinically significant cancer in the prostate is important for the precise focal therapy. Since February 2016, the biopsy with BioJet was approved as the advance medical technique by Japanese Ministry of Health, Labor, and Welfare.

3.2. The evaluation of the effectiveness and the local recurrence of the prostate cancer after the focal therapy with HIFU

The treated areas with HIFU in the prostate appear as nonenhanced areas on contrast-enhanced T1-weighted MRI, and subsequent transrectal biopsies have been able to remove homogenous necrotic tissue sections from the nonenhanced area [16]. Therefore, contrast-enhanced MRI has been considered to be the evaluation method of choice to demonstrate the effectiveness of HIFU for localized prostate cancer. We reported the time-dependent changes in blood flow within the prostate treated with HIFU on contrast-enhanced MRI between postoperative days 1 and 14 [16]. In addition, pathological analysis showed vessel damage with coagulative degeneration and detachment of vascular endothelial cells in HIFU-treated prostate tissue [16]. Previous studies [5] have shown that these time-dependent changes in blood flow within the prostate are likely due to the primary thermal effects induced on the tissue and vessel damage by coagulative degeneration in the prostate and that cavitation rapidly induces the detachment of vascular endothelial cells, gradually decreasing blood flow secondary to vessel obstruction. Future large-scale studies should investigate the most appropriate timing of contrast-enhanced MRI for precise feedback regarding the effectiveness of HIFU. Using the contrast-enhanced MRI, the evaluation of the effectiveness and the local recurrence of the prostate cancer needs to be evaluated after the focal therapy with HIFU.

4. The original protocol and the early experience of the focal therapy for the prostate cancer in our institution

Since 2016, the patients with low- and intermediate-risk group who were diagnosed the spatial localization of the prostate significant cancer in the prostate were recruited prospectively. The spatial localization of the significant cancer was diagnosed with MRI-transrectal ultrasound (TRUS) fusion image-guided transperineal prostate biopsy using the BioJet® system (D&K Technologies GmbH, Barum, Germany). The focal therapy was performed to the significant cancer detected regions with transrectal HIFU using Sonablate® 500 (SonaCare medical, Indianapolis, IN, USA). To evaluate the efficacy of the treatment, serum prostate-specific antigen (PSA) kinetics and three-dimensional (3D) reconstructed multiparametric MRI were analyzed (**Figure 1**). To evaluate the invasiveness, questionnaires (IPSS, QOL, OABSS, IIEF-5, SF-36 Japanese version 2) and uroflowmetry were performed. Adverse event was evaluated with Common Terminology Criteria for Adverse Events (CTCAE) ver.4.0. Fifteen patients with median age of 64 years (48–79) and median PSA of 7.2 ng/ml (4.67–15.99) were treated. All men (15 of 15 patients) had pad-free/leak-free continence at 1 and 3 months after the treatment. The proportion of men with erections sufficient for penetration was not changed from 73% (11 of 15 patients) to 73%. Catheterization was within 24 hours after the treatment in all patients. The median PSA of the patients significantly dropped from 7.2 to 1.76 ng/ml ($p = 0.001$) at 3 months after the treatment. The contrast-enhanced MRI and dynamic MRI showed the disappearance of blood flow in all targeted regions of the prostate with 3D evaluation of the MRI. There was no significant difference between before and after the treatment at 3 months in urinary symptoms (IPSS change, $p = 0.3$, QOL change $p = 0.7$, OABSS change, $p = 0.6$, max flow rate change, $p = 0.6$, residual urine change, $p = 0.1$), erectile function (IIEF-5 change, $p = 0.6$), and QOL (SF-36 change in all domains). Urinary tract infection with

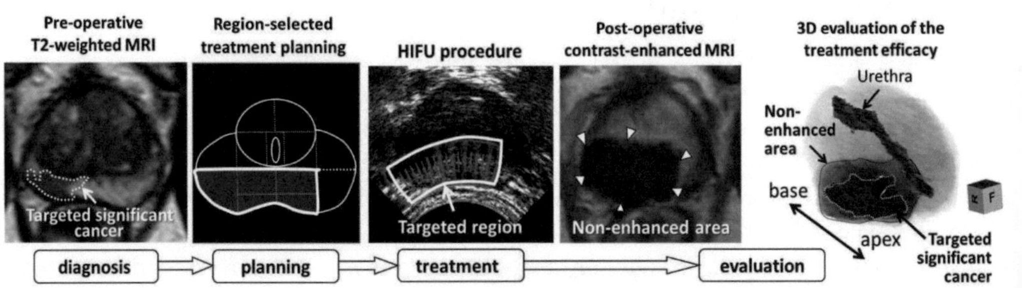

Figure 1. The protocol schema of focal HIFU treatment for the prostate cancer in our institution.

CTCAE Grade 2 was found in one patient (6.7%). In conclusion, the anatomical region selected focal therapy with HIFU would have potential to provide promising results with accurate treatment for the significant cancer and low morbidity.

5. Conclusion

MRI has the role of the management of the focal therapy with HIFU. Clinical trials have shown potential for effective focal treatment with HIFU-localized prostate cancer. Further oncological and functional outcomes in the patients treated with focal therapy with HIFU would be expected.

Acknowledgements

We like to offer our special thanks to Tomohisa Machida for creating pathological specimens and Akio Hashimoto and Tomoya Nakamura for MRI shooting in our institution.

Author details

Sunao Shoji[1]* and Akira Miyajima[2]

*Address all correspondence to: sunashoj@mail.goo.ne.jp

1 Department of Urology, Tokai University Hachioji Hospital, Tokyo, Japan

2 Department of Urology, Tokai University School of Medicine, Kanagawa, Japan

References

[1] Fry WJ, Barnard JW, Fry EJ, et al. Ultrasonic lesions in the mammalian central nervous system. Science. 1955;**122**:517-518

[2] Chapelon JY, Margonari J, Vernier F, et al. In vivo effects of high-intensity ultrasound on prostatic adenocarcinoma dunning R3327. Cancer Research. 1992;**52**:6353-6357

[3] Madersbacher S, Pedevilla M, Vingers L, et al. Effect of high-intensity focused ultrasound on human prostate cancer in vivo. Cancer Research. 1995;**55**:3346-3351

[4] Serrone J, Kocaeli H, Douglas Mast T, et al. The potential applications of high-intensity focused ultrasound (HIFU) in vascular neurosurgery. Journal of Clinical Neuroscience. 2012;**19**:214-221

[5] Wu F, Chen WZ, Bai J, et al. Pathological changes in human malignant carcinoma treated with high-intensity focused ultrasound. Ultrasound in Medicine & Biology. 2001;**27**:1099-1106

[6] Ahmed HU, Freeman A, Kirkham A, et al. Focal therapy for localized prostate cancer: A phase I/II trial. The Journal of Urology. 2011;**185**:1246-1254

[7] Ahmed HU, Hindley RG, Dickinson L, et al. Focal therapy for localised unifocal and multifocal prostate cancer: A prospective development study. The Lancet Oncology. 2012;**13**:622-632

[8] El Fegoun AB, Barret E, Prapotnich D, et al. Focal therapy with high-intensity focused ultrasound for prostate cancer in the elderly. A feasibility study with 10 years follow-up. International Brazilian Journal of Urology. 2011;**37**:213-219; discussion 220-2

[9] Muto S, Yoshii T, Saito K, et al. Focal therapy with high-intensity-focused ultrasound in the treatment of localized prostate cancer. Japanese Journal of Clinical Oncology. 2008;**38**: 192-199

[10] Shoji S, Nakano M, Fujikawa H, et al. Urethra-sparing high-intensity focused ultrasound for localized prostate cancer: Functional and oncological outcomes. International Journal of Urology. 2015;**22**:1043-1049

[11] Van Velthoven R, Aoun F, Limani K, et al. Primary zonal high intensity focused ultrasound for prostate cancer: Results of a prospective phase IIa feasibility study. Prostate Cancer. 2014;**2014**(756189)

[12] Moore CM, Kasivisvanathan V, Eggener S, et al. Standards of reporting for MRI-targeted biopsy studies (START) of the prostate: Recommendations from an international working group. European Urology. 2013;**64**:544-552

[13] Sciarra A, Panebianco V, Ciccariello M, et al. Value of magnetic resonance spectroscopy imaging and dynamic contrast-enhanced imaging for detecting prostate cancer foci in men with prior negative biopsy. Clinical Cancer Research. 2010;**16**:1875-1883

[14] Dickinson L, Ahmed HU, Allen C, et al. Magnetic resonance imaging for the detection, localisation, and characterisation of prostate cancer: Recommendations from a European consensus meeting. European Urology. 2011;**59**:477-494

[15] Shoji S, Hiraiwa S, Ogawa T, et al. Accuracy of real-time magnetic resonance imaging-transrectal ultrasound fusion image-guided transperineal target biopsy with needle tracking with a mechanical position-encoded stepper in detecting significant prostate cancer in biopsy-naive men. International Journal of Urology. 2017;**24**:288-294

[16] Shoji S, Tonooka A, Hashimoto A, et al. Time-dependent change of blood flow in the prostate treated with high-intensity focused ultrasound. International Journal of Urology. 2014;**21**:942-945

Chapter 3

3D Polarized Light Imaging Portrayed: Visualization of Fiber Architecture Derived from 3D-PLI

Nicole Schubert, Markus Axer, Uwe Pietrzyk and Katrin Amunts

Additional information is available at the end of the chapter

http://dx.doi.org/10.5772/intechopen.72532

Abstract

3D polarized light imaging (3D-PLI) is a neuroimaging technique that has recently opened up new avenues to study the complex architecture of nerve fibers in postmortem brains at microscopic scales. In a specific voxel-based analysis, each voxel is assigned a single 3D fiber orientation vector. This leads to comprehensive 3D vector fields. In order to inspect and analyze such high-resolution fiber orientation vector field, also in combination with complementary microscopy measurements, appropriate visualization techniques are essential to overcome several challenges, such as the massive data sizes, the large amount of both unique and redundant information at different scales, or the occlusion issues of inner structures by outer layers. Here, we introduce a comprehensive software tool that is able to visualize all information of a typical 3D-PLI dataset in an adequate and sophisticated manner. This includes the visualization of (i) anatomic structural and fiber architectonic data in one representation, (ii) a large-scale fiber orientation vector field, and (iii) a clustered version of the field. Alignment of a 3D-PLI dataset to an appropriate brain atlas provides expert-based delineation, segmentation, and, ultimately, visualization of selected anatomical structures. By means of these techniques, a detailed analysis of the complex fiber architecture in 3D is feasible.

Keywords: polarized light imaging, scientific visualization, neuroinformatics, neuroimaging and fiber architecture

1. Introduction

3D-PLI is an essential microscopy method that makes the derivation of 3D nerve fiber orientations possible [1–3]. It provides 3D fiber orientation models that are interpreted by a voxel-based analysis, i.e., each tissue voxel is assigned a single 3D fiber orientation vector. The 3D reconstruction of images of serial brain section by means of image registration yields a virtual brain model reflecting local fiber orientations. The unique value of 3D-PLI data was demonstrated in detailed studies of the course of fibers and fiber tracts in section-wise 3D analysis [4, 5], i.e., the fibers were traced across the sections by means of 2D visualizations. A structural analysis of fiber orientation models in 3D requires specific visualization techniques due to the challenges the 3D visualization of fiber architecture is confronted with, such as the huge amount of data, the occlusion of the inner structures by the outer layers, and the visual clutter caused by the enormous number of vectors contained in the datasets.

In this chapter, we will introduce 3D visualization techniques that extract important information of the 3D-PLI data and present them appropriately. First, the method of 3D-PLI is briefly summarized including the tissue processing, image acquisition, and image processing. The methods that are used to visualize our fiber orientation models are illustrated as well as the structural modalities that will be needed as anatomical context. In addition examples are presented of how these techniques can be used to trace the 3D courses of fibers in 3D in human and rat brains. As such new methods are provided for quantitative 3D analysis of the fiber architecture of mammalian brains.

2. 3D polarized light imaging in a nutshell

The polarization microscopy technology referred to as 3D-PLI is able to reveal the brain's fiber architecture at the micro- to the mesoscale (i.e., in the range of 1–100 μm) in serial large-sized unstained histological brain sections [1–5]. 3D-PLI demonstrated exceptional performance in providing fiber/non-fiber contrasts in both deep white matter and cortical regions even for entire human brain sections with an area size of up to 200 cm^2 scanned at very high spatial resolution (down to 1.3 μm, in-plane). No histological staining or labeling is needed by optical methods that utilize intrinsic tissue properties able to modify the polarization state of light. Birefringence, the main polarization property of interest for biological tissues, is caused by a difference in index of refraction that results in a phase shift between orthogonal polarization states and is often exhibited by fibrous structures, such as nerve fibers (i.e., myelinated and unmyelinated axons). 3D-PLI utilizes the birefringence of myelinated and to a minor extent also unmyelinated axons in histological sections to contrast fibers with nerve cell bodies or glial cells and to determine their spatial courses in a form of 3D fiber orientation vectors. Apparently, 3D-PLI images disclose an intriguing fiber architecture, which integrates classic myeloarchitecture [6] with tissue anisotropy as revealed by diffusion magnetic resonance imaging on a microscopic level [3, 5, 7, 8]. 3D-PLI has an obvious important bridging function between the macroscopic and the microscopic world of fiber architecture, i.e., between fiber pathways and single fibers.

3D-PLI involves the preparation of histological brain sections, their imaging with polarimetric setups, the calculation of fiber orientations based on a physical model, and the section realignment with subsequent data interpretation as briefly described in the following.

2.1. Tissue sectioning and block face imaging

The entire brains of an adult human or a rat were immersion fixed in 4% buffered formaldehyde. After two cryoprotection steps (10% glycerine for 3 days, followed by 20% glycerine for

14 days at +4°C), the brains were deep frozen in isopentane at −50°C and serially sectioned in the coronal, sagittal, or horizontal plane at 60 μm thickness using cryostat microtomes (Leica Microsystems, Germany). The ensuing sections were placed on glass slides and stored at −80°C in airtight plastic bags until further processing. They were thaw mounted and coverslipped with 20% glycerine the day before image acquisition took place. Note that there was no staining applied to the tissue, since the imaging technique 3D-PLI solely relies on intrinsic optical properties. The results of the procedure are sequential series of sections of complete brains. During sectioning of the brain, block face images of every section were taken with a CCD camera (AVT Oscar F-810 C, 3272 × 2469 pixels, 15 μm × 15 μm, RGB) which was installed vertically above the cryostat. 3D alignment of the block face images (cf. Section 2.4) yields an undistorted reference brain volume essential for both 3D histological reconstruction and visualization.

2.2. Image acquisition

Two polarimetric devices are used to address complementary scales to study fiber architecture: the large area polarimeter (LAP) and the polarizing microscope (PM) [1–3]. The LAP enables a single-shot imaging of whole human brain sections at 64 μm pixel size in-plane covering a field of view with a diameter of up to 20 cm. The PM covers a much smaller field of view (2.7 mm × 2.7 mm) but provides 1.3 μm pixel size in-plane. In order to scan large areas with the PM, a motorized scanning stage has been built into the microscope, which acquires entire section images in tiles. The tiles have to be stichted together during post processing. The general optical setup used in the LAP is shown in **Figure 1(a)**, in which the specimen is sandwiched between two linear polarization filters with orthogonal transmission axes and a quarter-wave retarder. A customized LED light source provides homogeneous green wavelength

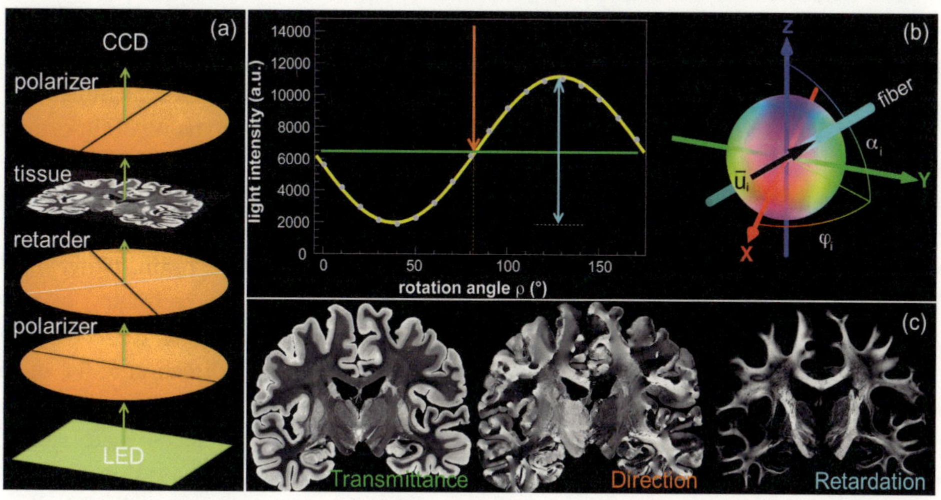

Figure 1. The polarimetric setup of 3D-PLI: A LED light source illuminates the brain section located between two linear polarizers and a quarter-wave retarder (a). The simultaneous rotation of the filters changes the signal captured by a CCD camera depending on the fiber orientation in each voxel of the section. The signal follows a sinusoidal course (b, left) and indicates the fiber angles (b, right) as well as the transmittance of the light (horizontal green line in (b, left), left in (c)), the direction of the fiber (orange arrow in (b, left), center in (c)), and the retardation (blue range in (b, left), right in (c)).

illumination. During simultaneous optical filter rotation, the intensity of the transmitted light varies strongly in a sinusoidal manner (**Figure 1(b)**), depending on the orientations of the underlying fibers or fiber tracts, respectively. This effect is caused by the nerve fibers' birefringence. The light intensities are measured at discrete angles in the range from 0 to 180° by a CCD camera (AxioCam HRc Rev.2, Zeiss, Germany) dedicated to microscopic imaging (see **Figure 1**).

2.3. 3D-PLI modalities

The measured sinusoidal signal (per image pixel) is interpreted by fitting a physical model derived from the Jones calculus [9] to it, as described in [1] (**Figure 1(b)** and **(c)**). This allows retrieving information about the light retardation, the light transmittance, and the fiber direction angle φ and inclination angle α reflecting the orientation of a fiber in 3D. The retardation is derived from the relative amplitude of the sinusoidal signal and encodes the local birefringence strength together with the fiber (out-of-section) inclination angle. The transmittance represents the mean value of the sinusoidal signal and describes the amount of light transmitted through the tissue, reduced by absorption and scattering processes. The fiber (in-plane) direction angle is defined by the phase of the sinusoidal signal. Both direction and inclination angles are combined to fiber orientation vectors building the fiber orientation maps (FOMs) for each brain section. A 3D fiber orientation model is generated by a 3D reconstruction of the maps. Note that FOMs represent vector-like data, while all other 3D-PLI modalities are scalar-valued data types.

2.4. 3D reconstruction

Nonlinear deformations introduced by brain sectioning and mounting are corrected using block face images as undistorted references for the spatial alignment of the 3D-PLI modalities [10]. In the first step, the block face images have to be 3D reconstructed. Briefly, the block face reconstruction method consists of a two-phase registration: a marker-based alignment of the images and a median-based refinement of the pre-reconstructed volume using 3D information. First, the coordinates of markers (ARTag, a marker adopted from augmented reality) labeled on the microtome chuck are extracted and aligned to the corresponding markers in the neighboring images by means of a translation transformation. Processing all images leads to an almost smoothly reconstructed 3D stack of block face images of the brain. However, this approach causes perspective errors due to the different heights of the sectioning plane and microtome chuck with the markers and thus their different distances to the camera lens. Therefore, in the second part of the method, the median along the z-direction of the marker-based reconstructed block face volume is calculated to eliminate the outliers caused by perspective errors. The marker-based reconstructed volume is aligned slice-by-slice onto the median volume using a translation transform estimated by an intensity based image registration algorithm. This technique takes advantage of 3D information in an actually 2D slice-by-slice registration method. This leads to an accurately aligned volume of block face images that serves as an important reference to recover the spatial coherence of the nonlinearly deformed sections corresponding to the block face images.

The 3D reconstruction of the 3D-PLI data consists of two steps: a rigid slice-by-slice registration of the 3D-PLI images to the corresponding block face images and a nonrigid refinement method. The first step is based on estimating a transformation of the 3D-PLI images to the corresponding image of the reconstructed block face volume by image registration. To align the 3D-PLI images to the block face images, the masks of the brain tissue of both datasets are required. A 3D watershed algorithm is used to segment the reconstructed block face volume, while the 3D-PLI images are segmented manually. Using the segmented images, the centers of gravity of the corresponding brain masks are calculated and aligned. Based on this initial transformation, an intensity-based rigid registration is performed. The second step, the refinement, is performed by a slice-by-slice B-spline registration yielding to 3D reconstructions of all 3D-PLI modalities.

2.5. Brain models

The techniques applied for visualization were investigated on two datasets, one rat brain and one human brain. All animal procedures were approved by the institutional animal welfare committee at the Research Centre of Jülich and were in accordance with the European Union (National Institutes of Health) guidelines for the use and care of laboratory animals. The human brain was acquired in accordance with local legal and ethical requirements.

The entire rat brain and one hemisphere of the human brain were serially cut and have been fully processed with both LAP and PM. The rat brain was sectioned into 455 sections of 60 μm thickness. The hemisphere of the human brain was cut from anterior to posterior along the coronal sectioning plane in 843 sections with a thickness of 70 μm. The generated 3D reconstructed fiber orientation model of the rat consists of a vector field with a size of 588 × 723 × 413 voxels and a resolution of 64 μm × 64 μm × 60 μm (LAP). The human hemisphere has a reconstructed vector field of 1350 × 1950 × 228 voxels and a voxel size of 64 μm × 64 μm × 70 μm (LAP).

In addition, the rat brain was spatially aligned to a common rat brain atlas, the Waxholm Space (WHS) atlas of the Sprague Dawley® rat brain [11, 12]. The three-dimensional atlas is publicly accessible and provided by the International Neuroinformatics Coordinating Facility (INCF) Software Center. The atlas is based on high-resolution MRI and DTI datasets of the brain of the Sprague Dawley rat anchored in the Waxholm Space and the stereotaxic space. The T2*-weighted anatomical MRI (512 × 1024 × 512 pixels) with isotropic local resolution of 39 μm was acquired ex vivo with a 7 T small animal MRI system. The DTI dataset has an isotropic spatial resolution of 79 μm. The anatomical boundaries in the atlas were drawn manually based on the image contrast of the T2*-weighted and DTI images. The latest version of the atlas contains 79 structures, including new and updated boundaries of the hippocampus and parahippocampus [13].

3. Visualization

The visualization techniques described here include both well-known methods of volume rendering and methods specifically developed for 3D-PLI, which in combination open up a new way of exploring the high-resolution fiber architecture. The techniques can be classified on the basis of the underlying data, since different visualization methods are required for the different types of data. 3D-PLI provides scalar and vector fields. A scalar field is a dataset with a scalar value per voxel, such as all 3D-PLI gray value modalities, while a vector field contains one vector per voxel, as in the fiber orientation model.

The scalar data are visualized using classic volume rendering techniques introduced in Section 3.1. The procedures have been implemented for interactive work on the graphics card. In addition, various features have been investigated which allow visualizing several volumes simultaneously. This enables an analysis of the complete dataset at the same time. The intuitive visualization of the vector fields, i.e., each vector as a line, has to overcome various difficulties, such as the occlusion of inner structures, visual clutter, and a slow performance of the visualization for larger datasets. The different ways of handling these challenges are presented in Section 3.2.

3.1. Visualization of 3D-PLI gray value maps

For the 3D representation of the gray value maps, existing 3D visualization techniques (volume rendering) can be used. Volume rendering is classified into indirect and direct rendering. Indirect volume rendering is based on the visualization of a previously calculated surface model. This model is a mesh of polygons, ideally a triangle mesh, as graphics cards are optimized to visualize those. The surface is determined by suitable methods. The best-known method is Marching cubes [14]. Direct volume rendering techniques construct a voxel model based on the underlying data that represents the object. Each voxel is assigned a color and transparency. Texture-based methods are very fast, but the more computationally intensive method ray casting is more flexible in terms of coloring [15]. Since the grayscale modalities in combination with the fiber model are primarily intended to be used as anatomical context, the coloring of the data is not essential. Therefore, we are focusing on the fast texture-based method texture slicing.

3.1.1. Surface rendering

Marching cubes calculates a triangle mesh that represents the surface of an object, based on a threshold t, the so-called isovalue. The algorithm marches through the entire volume along the voxels and forms a cube with eight voxels each (**Figure 2(a)**). The gray values at the edges of the cube are then compared with t. Here, three different cases can occur: (i) all values are below t, i.e., the complete cube does not belong to the object; (ii) all values are above t, i.e., the complete cube belongs to the object; or (iii) some values are above, some below t. In the latter case, the surface is defined by a set of triangles which separates the vertices that are larger than t, i.e., belong to the object, from the other vertices that are not belonging to the object. After the entire dataset is traversed, a complete triangle mesh is created. The triangular mesh filled with a certain color can then be efficiently visualized by optimized algorithms provided by the graphics card. In addition the illumination of the scene also plays an important role. For the combined visualization with the fiber orientation model, it is important that the surface is visualized transparently (**Figure 2(b)**). In order to accelerate the calculation of the surface mesh, it was transferred to the graphics card.

3.1.2. Volume rendering

In texture slicing, a volumetric dataset is visualized as a stack of parallel sections arranged next to each other. A 3D texture is created in the graphics card, which contains the volume. Parallel to the image plane, a stack of 2D textures is generated through the volume. The 2D textures are filled with scalar values by means of trilinear interpolation of the 3D texture containing the volume. Color and opacity can be set by color tables. Texture slicing also takes advantage of the hardware-near implementation, as the graphics cards are designed for the fast use of texture memory and the computation-intensive interpolations are accelerated on the graphics card. In order to reveal the inner structures of the volumes and also to be able to combine the visualization with further data, clipping boxes must be used in texture slicing, which interactively remove areas of the object (**Figure 3**).

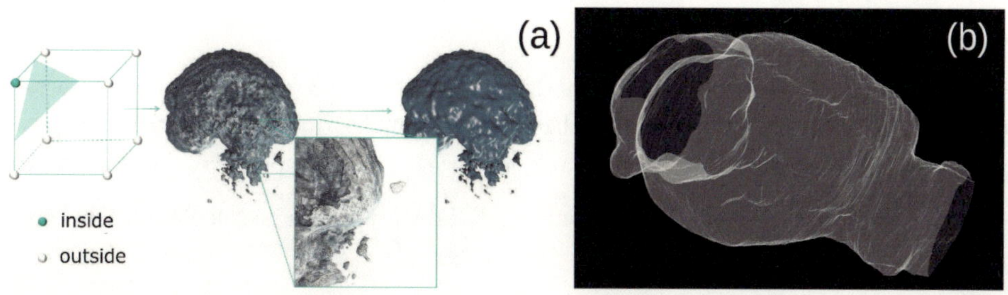

Figure 2. Surface rendering with Marching cubes. The volume is traversed by a cube of eight voxels (a). Each voxel of the cube is inspected whether its value is inside or outside the surface. The cube is divided into triangles that form a triangle mesh. The triangle mesh can then be visualized filled with a color and suitable illumination. A transparent interface is very useful to provide a visual context for a combined visualization including further data (b).

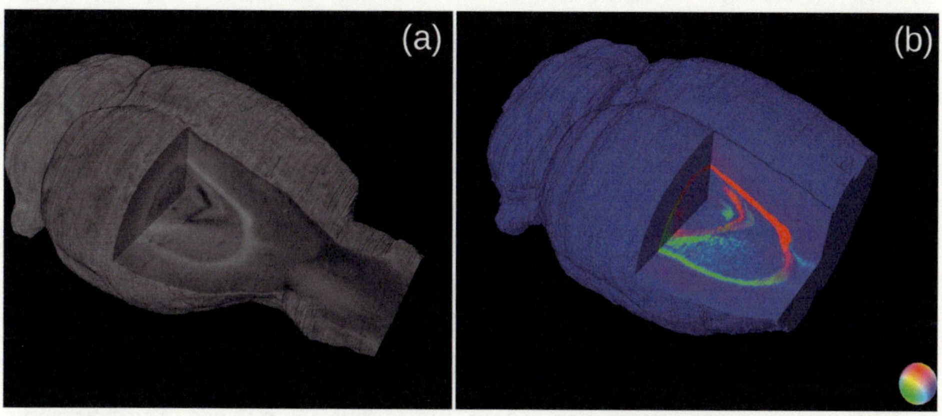

Figure 3. Volume rendering with texture slicing. With the help of maneuverable and scalable boxes, the internal structures of the gray value visualization (a) as well as the colored visualization (b) become visible.

3.2. Visualization of the 3D fiber orientation model

A 3D fiber orientation model is a 3D vector field that represents the fiber orientation per voxel. A direct way to visualize a vector field is to use glyphs [16]. Glyphs are small geometric objects that can represent different properties of the vectors by their color and shape, such as position, direction, orientation, and size. A variable and fast method to calculate glyphs is presented in Section 3.2.1. The color is an important factor as it can indicate certain properties such as the direction of the vectors (Section 3.2.2).

The visualization of the fiber orientation of an entire brain by glyphs is opaque and thus inaccessible for analysis. The outer layers occlude the inner structures. Therefore, suitable methods have been developed that provide an insight into the vector field and thus into the fiber architecture of the brain. This includes the combined visualization with an anatomical dataset (Section 3.2.3), the clustering of vectors to a more bundled visualization (Section 3.2.4), and the visualization of the vectors as nerve fiber pathways (Section 3.2.5). In addition, a 3D atlas can be used for visualization beyond the scope of an anatomical context, as shown in Section 3.2.6.

3.2.1. Glyphs

For each voxel of the fiber orientation model, the position and orientation of the vector are extracted. Each vector can then be visualized as a geometric form with variable length and width. By means of the voxel coordinate, which serves as starting point $\overrightarrow{p_{start}}$ of the glyph and the orientation $\vec{d}$ of the vector, an end point pend of the glyph can be calculated. The length of the vector l is variable in the range [0, 1]:

$$\overrightarrow{p_{end}} = \overrightarrow{p_{start}} + l \cdot \vec{d} \tag{1}$$

The two points can be used to define an undirected line per voxel and to represent the fiber orientation vector. A line represents the position and orientation of a vector. However, in a 3D vector field, the distances of the vectors to each other and the occlusions of the vectors are difficult to distinguish. A 3D shape of the glyphs significantly improves the spatial impression of the 3D vector field. Thus, glyph positions and distances between the glyphs can be clearly recognized. A cylinder is the most suitable glyph shape as it models the round shape of the nerve fibers. In computer graphics, circles (the base of a cylinder) are approximated, in which points on the real circle are calculated and connected with the smallest possible distance. The parametric equation of a circle can be used for this purpose:

$$\vec{r}\,(\vartheta) = \begin{pmatrix} x(\vartheta) \\ y(\vartheta) \end{pmatrix} = \begin{pmatrix} r \cdot \cos\vartheta \\ r \cdot \sin\vartheta \end{pmatrix} \tag{2}$$

with $\vartheta \epsilon [0, 2\pi]$ and the radius r.

Since this is computationally very demanding, considering the millions of vectors and thus cylinders that have to be calculated, the base areas of the glyphs are defined only by a few points (vertices). For example, a cuboid has four vertices, and the cylinder to be represented has six vertices. The number of vertices can be set individually which provides space for higher-resolution circles.

The vertices v_i around the start and end point of the glyphs are now calculated as follows (**Figure 4**). The number of vertices n determines the angular distance between the vertices on the circle:

$$\vartheta = (2 \cdot \pi)/n \tag{3}$$

With the help of this angle and the parametric equation of a circle, the vertices v_i can be described:

$$\overrightarrow{v_{i_s}} = \overrightarrow{p_{start}} + \vec{d} \begin{pmatrix} r \cdot \cos\vartheta \\ r \cdot \sin\vartheta \\ 0 \end{pmatrix} \text{ resp. } \overrightarrow{v_{i_e}} = \overrightarrow{p_{end}} + \vec{d} \begin{pmatrix} r \cdot \cos\vartheta \\ r \cdot \sin\vartheta \\ 0 \end{pmatrix} \tag{4}$$

Before the coordinates are added to the start or end point, they must be multiplied by the vector orientation $\vec{d}$ to avoid displaying the glyph as oblique prism.

The length and width of the glyphs can be set interactively by changing the variables r and l. Another important aspect is the color coding of the glyphs, which is another visual indicator for the orientation of the fibers. Thus, fibers with the same orientations are directly recognizable and visually discriminable from other orientations.

3.2.2. *Color coding and lighting*

Two color spaces are used for the color coding of the glyphs, RGB and HSV. The RGB color space is an additive color space based on the three primary colors red, green, and blue. The x, y, and z components of the vector orientation are assigned directly to the three basic colors, i.e., the x-direction is encoded in red, the y-direction in green, and the z-direction in blue. The HSV color space defines color by the color value hue ([0, 360]), the color saturation ([0, 1]), and the brightness value ([0, 1]). The color value is determined by the x- and y-component of the vector, the z-component influences the brightness of the color, and the saturation is set to the

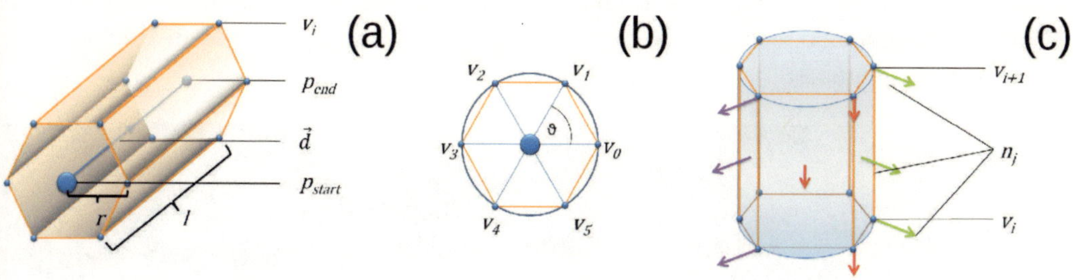

Figure 4. To calculate the glyph, the voxel coordinate (blue circle) is used as starting point $\overrightarrow{p_{start}}$, and the orientation of the vector $\vec{d}$ is used to determine an end point $\overrightarrow{p_{end}}$ (a). The variable l specifies the length of the glyph. The shape of the glyph is defined with a given radius r and a number of vertices v_i. The angle ϑ determines the distance between the vertices (b). Using the example of six vertices as shown in the picture, the angle is 60°. To calculate the surface normals, vertices v_i and v_{i+1} are assigned the normal vector n_j, where j is the number of the current rectangle (c).

maximum 1. For this purpose, the two angles are calculated from the vector components by means of spherical coordinates:

$$\varphi = \arctan\left(\frac{y}{x}\right), \quad \alpha = \arcsin(z) \tag{5}$$

and then the color can be calculated:

$$H = 2\cdot\varphi, \quad S = 1 - \frac{\alpha}{90^{\circ}}, \quad V = 1 \tag{6}$$

Color-coded representations of the fiber orientation can be found in **Figure 5**. The color spheres serve as a legend. In the HSV space (**Figure 5(b)**), symmetric orientations can be better distinguished in the plane than in the RGB space (**Figure 5(a)**). For example, yellow in the RGB space codes orientations that run diagonally from the bottom left or bottom right, while these orientations in the HSV space are represented by the different colors green and blue. In order to emphasize the colors of the vectors in the plane, the saturation and value channel are swapped so that the vectors running perpendicular to the plane are visualized in black instead of white (**Figure 5(c)**). This generates a special HSV color scheme (HSV black).

To better recognize the 3D structures, lights are used which darken the colors inside the glyphs by creating shadows. To distinguish between inside and outside the glyphs, the surface normals have to be calculated. For each rectangle that approximates the cylinder, one surface normal is calculated using the cross product. This surface normal is assigned to the first two points of the rectangle (**Figure 4(c)**). The other two points are used to calculate the next normal. This produces continuous shading as a form of the local lighting model Gouraud shading [17].

3.2.3. *Combined visualization*

To get an insight into a 3D vector field, clipping boxes are needed [18]. A clipping box defines a region that is excluded from the visualization in order to reveal the underlying information. The offset and the size of the box can be interactively changed. In order to obtain an anatomical context despite the removal of vector information, it is an advantage to additionally visualize a PLI modality by means of volume rendering. This means that either the surface of the brain (**Figure 6(a)**) or the entire volume as 3D texture (**Figure 6(b)**) can be visualized together with the clipped fiber orientation model. In the case of 3D textures, two clipping boxes are used to mask out the regions of interest.

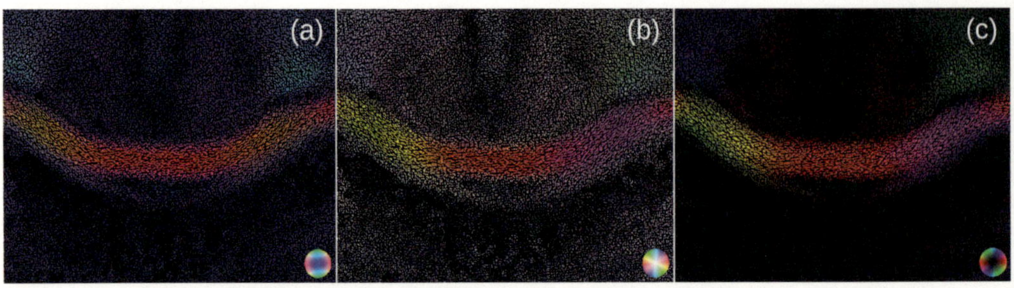

Figure 5. The color-coded glyphs are shown in the RGB color space (a), in the HSV color space (b), and in a special HSV color space: HSV black (c). The colored spheres in the lower right corner of every image are used as legends.

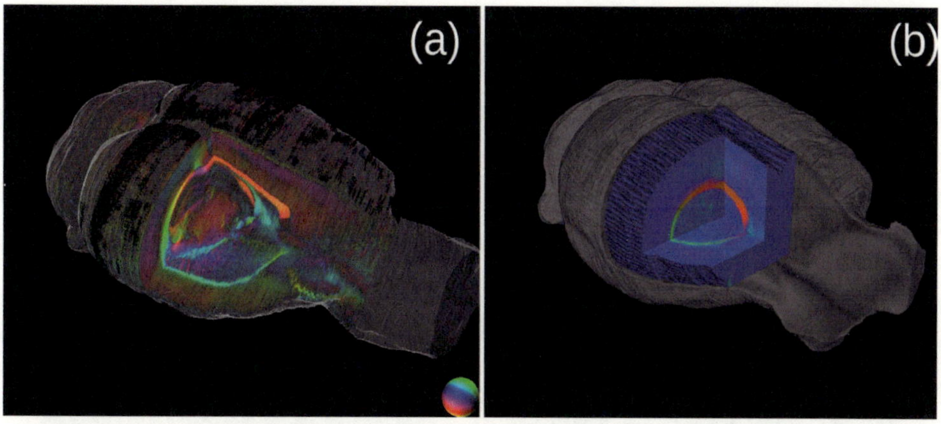

Figure 6. In order to get an insight into the brain, clipping boxes are used to remove parts of the brain. For an anatomical context, structural data are visualized as surface (a) and as 3D texture (b) in combination with the fiber orientation model.

3.2.4. Clustering of fiber orientations

The 3D fiber orientation model contains very dense information, one vector per voxel. Consequently, the visualization is also very dense. Therefore, the visualization may contain too much information; hence, it might not be possible for the viewer to figure out the important information. A reduction of the information can help to get a better overview of all orientations in the model. A quick way of reducing information is to remove every x-th vector from the visualization, but this may also lead to the loss of important information. A better option is to group directions [7, 19]. The fiber orientation model is divided into cuboids of equal size, so-called super-voxels. For each super-voxel region, a 3D histogram is created, which calculates the frequency of the orientations of the vectors in the super-voxel. For this purpose, a unit sphere is divided into bins, i.e., in the case of a sphere, degrees of longitude and latitude. The best match of an orientation vector is determined by the maximum scalar product with the central vector of every bin of the sphere. With the help of the histogram, a direction can now be displayed by super-voxel, using the same algorithms as described in Section 2.2.1. **Figure 7** shows a section of the human hemisphere visualized with different super-voxel sizes, showing there is no notable loss of information. In order to ensure that no information is lost, it is possible to display the strongest directions in super-voxel up to a defined number at the same time. This means that no information is lost even at sharp transitions between fiber orientations. In addition, the vector field can be displayed as an information source (**Figure 8**). Thus, an overall impression of the orientations in the model is easily obtained without significant loss of information.

3.2.5. Fiber pathways

The analysis of fiber architecture implies the visualization of nerve fiber pathways. For this purpose, the pathways have to be reconstructed from the vector field before they can be visualized. The reconstruction of the fiber pathways is a comprehensive and complex task that has been intensively studied for DTI data [20–22], but not yet in depth for 3D-PLI data. Nevertheless, some algorithms can be adapted. We use a deterministic algorithm for the

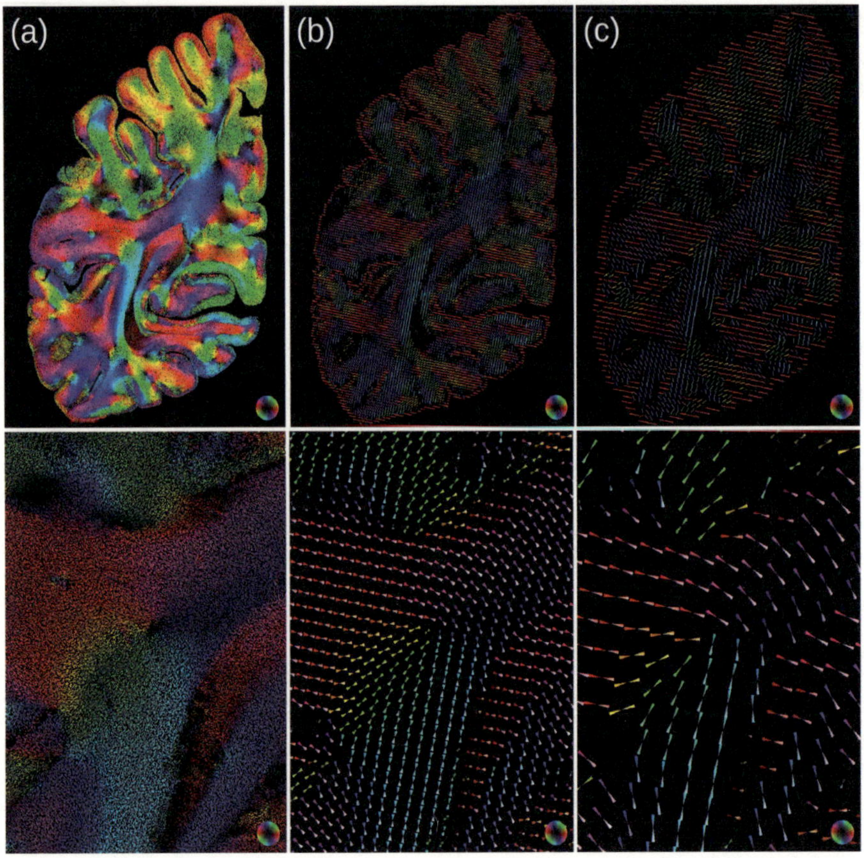

Figure 7. One section of the human hemisphere visualized with one line per vector (a) and two clustered vector fields with one line per super-voxel with super-voxels containing 10×10×1 vectors (b) and 20×20×1 vectors (c). A detailed view is located at the bottom of each section. The decrease of the resolution by increasing the super-voxel size shows no significant loss of information.

3D-PLI data, which propagates through the vector field from different starting points (seed points) and thus identifies possible fiber pathways [20].

Mathematically, propagating through the vector field from one seed point can be considered as solving an initial value problem using numerical methods. Common linear methods to solve initial value problems are the Euler and Runge-Kutta methods. Both methods start at a seed point. With a defined step size, the propagator moves in the direction of the vector of the seed point. At the new point, the new direction is determined by means of interpolation, and propagation continues until the end of the vector field is reached. The Runge-Kutta method uses additional intermediate steps to calculate the new direction. This is why the Runge-Kutta method is more computation-intensive but more accurate as compared to the Euler method.

The tractography of the 3D-PLI vector field results in a list of points describing the fiber paths. For each given seed point, the possible paths through the vector field are approximated. Since the 3D-PLI data do not provide direction but orientation, the vector field is traversed in both directions. The tractography is terminated as soon as the path leaves the vector field or the area

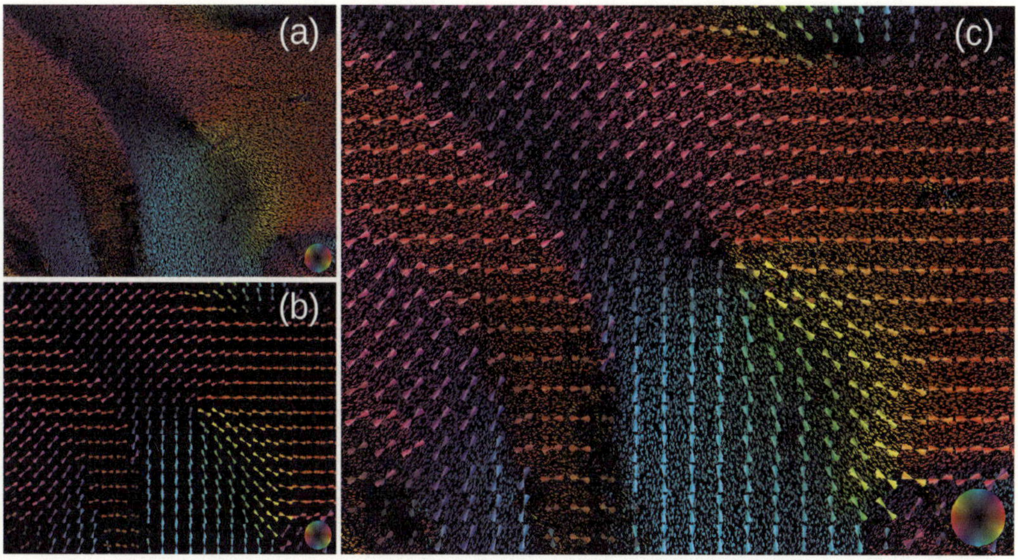

Figure 8. Detailed visualization of the human hemisphere: (a) the 3D vector field, (b) the vector field after clustering the data with a super-voxel containing 10×10×1 vectors and visualized as pyramidal glyphs with the three strongest directions in the super-voxel, and (c) the combined visualization of the super-voxel glyphs with the underlying vector field.

to be viewed or a user-defined number of path points is reached. In addition, a maximum angle difference serves as a stop criterion. The calculations are performed in parallel for each seed point. A challenge in the tractography procedures is the setting of the initial values or seed points. If each voxel of the volume is used as a seed point, the results will quickly become confusing and difficult to evaluate. If only subregions are considered, one misses possible connections. Neuroanatomical knowledge is essential for the manual placement of seed points. Interactive setting of seed points, e.g., by cuboids, with subsequent visualization of the fiber pathways, facilitates revealing interesting pathways. Another anatomically based method for seed placement is the integration of 3D-PLI data into an anatomical atlas (Section 2.2.6). Here, the existing structures of the atlas can be used to use anatomically based seed points (**Figure 9**).

The reconstructed nerve fiber pathways are given as a list of linked points. The easiest way to visualize these paths is to display them as lines. A better impression of depth is achieved by using 3D shapes such as ribbons or tubes. For this representation, the same algorithm can be used to display the vector glyphs (Section 2.2.1). A circle is approximated around each fiber point by calculating vertices on a real circle. The circle points calculated per point are then connected to form ribbons or tubes. To enable a smooth surface also at the intermediate points at sharp curves, the position of the circle points is interpolated between the fiber sections. The length of the glyphs is defined by the distance between the fiber points; only the radius r is variable. The color coding as well as the lighting is equivalent to that of the glyphs (Section 2.2.2).

3.2.6. Anatomical region-based visualization

In order to ensure an anatomical region-based visualization, it is necessary to separate the brain regions from each other. This is usually done by a neuroanatomical expert using a 2D atlas to correlate to the 2D layers of the data. For 3D data, an extensive post-processing of the selections in the other cutting planes is necessary. This task is very time-consuming, labor-intensive, and prone to intra- and interobserver variability. A more recent approach transforms the datasets into a reference space that is ideally stereotactically standardized, e.g., in the Paxinos coordinate system [23].

We aligned a complete 3D-PLI rat brain dataset with the Waxholm Space atlas of the Sprague Dawley rat brain [11]. In order to ensure an accurate analysis of the 3D-PLI data, the atlas data were transformed into the coordinate space of the reconstructed data using advanced image registration algorithms [12]. The delineated regions of the atlas can be used to create an atlas-based visualization. The regions in the atlas are used as masks, so that only information of the selected regions is visible. This can be applied to all available modalities.

Once an anatomical region has been selected, the complex fiber architecture, represented, for example, by the fiber orientation glyphs, can be investigated and viewed in real time under

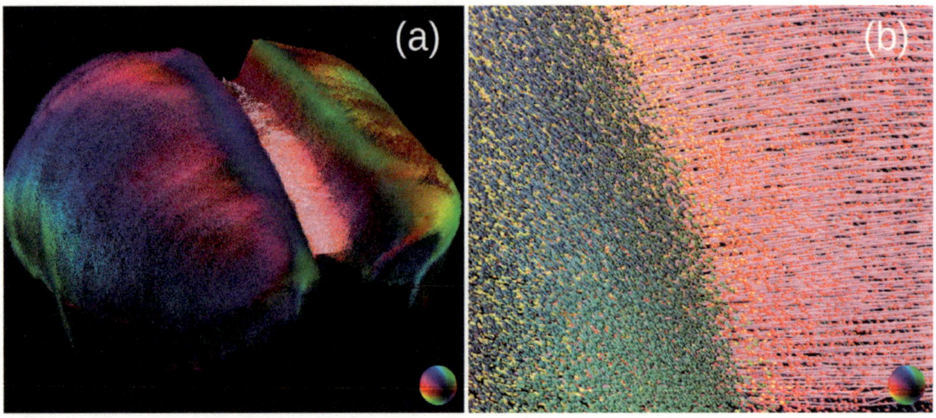

Figure 9. Fiber pathways (magenta) provided by tractography inside the corpus callosum of the rat brain with seed points on the midsagittal plane visualized together with the 3D vector field of the corpus callosum (a). Mainly, fiber pathways connecting the hemispheres can be seen (b).

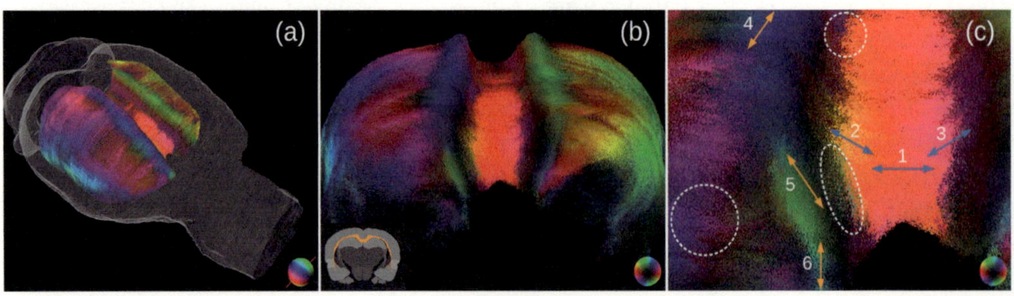

Figure 10. Using an atlas facilitates an anatomical region-based visualization, for instance, of the corpus callosum of the rat brain (a). Interactions with the model enable a visual analysis in all directions (b). Zooming into the fiber orientation model unveils different orientations and interrelations (c), left to right (arrow 1), lower right to upper left (arrows 2 and 5), lower left to upper right (arrows 3 and 4), and from top to bottom (arrow 6). The circles point to diverse sites, where fiber orientations are perpendicular to each other. This indicates regions with fibers running orthogonal to the image plane.

different viewing angles and magnification by rotation, translation, and zooming as demonstrated for the corpus callosum (**Figure 10**). The displayed fiber orientations unveil the complex network of fibers and fiber bundles in the corpus callosum. The visualization tool shows that the orientation of fibers in the corpus callosum is not restricted to bundles running in parallel in the midline region, and then fanning out, but rather shows an architecture with partly abrupt changes in orientation (**Figure 10**, arrows) and fibers crossing the corpus callosum orthogonally, including regions close to the midline (**Figure 10**, circles).

In addition, the present method enabled overcoming the problem of visual clutter and tangle. By masking out the structures of interest, the amount of data to visualize has been reduced, which allows to study fiber orientations interactively. Due to the option to use clipping boxes also in the regions of interest, a precise and high-resolution investigation of the fiber architecture has become feasible.

4. Conclusions and future perspectives

The developed methods resulted in a comprehensive tool that allows a detailed and high-resolution 3D exploration of the fiber architecture based on the fiber orientation models derived from 3D-PLI. Clipping planes reveal the fiber architecture of the model. By adding further modalities and their visualization as surface or volume to the model, an anatomical context is provided. The additional clustering of 3D-PLI vectors or the tracing of fiber paths from the vector field reduces visual clutter and enables interactive work with the data. By clustering the high-resolution data, the 3D-PLI data can be compared to DTI data, despite DTI provides a lower resolution than 3D-PLI [7]. 3D-PLI-based vector-type datasets are essential prerequisites for comprehensive fiber tractography at high spatial resolution, which will be investigated in future projects. The use of atlas-based parcellations represents a powerful approach not only to interpret the topography of fibers but also to improve visualization in anatomical regions of interest. The visualization techniques enable new insights into the complex fiber architecture of the brain and unveil the different orientations and interrelations of fibers and fiber bundles (**Figure 11**).

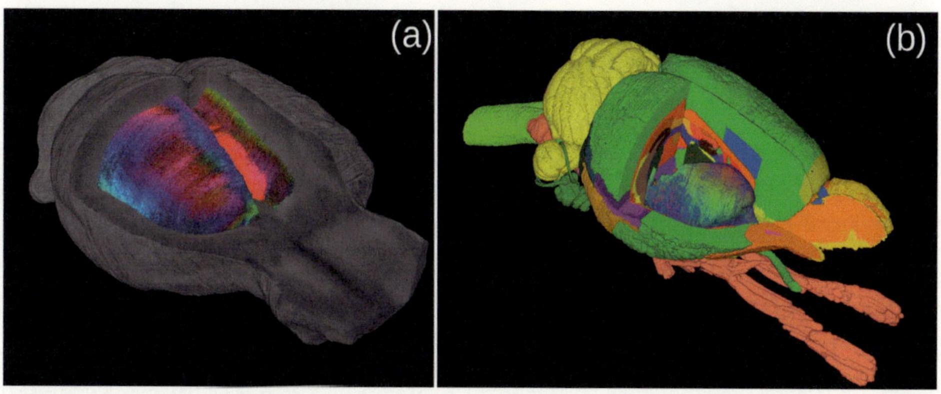

Figure 11. The atlas-based visualization of the fiber orientation model is also possible in combination with a 3D-PLI texture (a) or the atlas delineation itself (b).

Acknowledgements

We would like to thank M. Cremer, Research Centre of Jülich, Germany, for her excellent technical assistance and preparation of the histological sections.

This study was partially supported by the National Institutes of Health under Grant Agreement No. R01MH092311, by the Helmholtz Association of German Research Centres through the Helmholtz Portfolio Theme "Supercomputing and Modelling for the Human Brain," and by the European Union's Horizon 2020 Research and Innovation Programme under Grant Agreement No. 7202070 (HBP SGA1).

The authors gratefully acknowledge the computing time granted by the John von Neumann Institute for Computing (NIC) and provided on the supercomputer JURECA at Jülich Supercomputing Centre (JSC).

Author details

Nicole Schubert[1]*, Markus Axer[1], Uwe Pietrzyk[1,2] and Katrin Amunts[1,3]

*Address all correspondence to: n.schubert@fz-juelich.de

1 Institutes of Neuroscience and Medicine (INM-1, INM-4), Research Centre Jülich, Jülich, Germany

2 Faculty of Mathematics and Natural Sciences, University of Wuppertal, Wuppertal, Germany

3 C. and O. Vogt Institute for Brain Research, Heinrich-Heine University Düsseldorf, Düsseldorf, Germany

References

[1] Axer M, Amunts K, Gräßel D, Palm C, Dammers J, Axer H, et al. A novel approach to the human connectome: Ultra-high resolution mapping of fiber tracts in the brain. NeuroImage. 2011;**54**:1091-1101. DOI: 10.1016/j.neuroimage.2010.08.075

[2] Axer M, Gräßel D, Kleiner M, Dammers J, Dickscheid T, Reckfort J, et al. High-resolution fiber tract reconstruction in the human brain by means of polarized light imaging (3D-PLI). Frontiers in Neuroinformatics. 2011;**5**:34. DOI: 10.3389/fninf.2011.00034

[3] Reckfort J, Wiese H, Pietrzyk U, Zilles K, Amunts K, Axer M. A multiscale approach for the reconstruction of the fiber architecture of the human brain based on 3D-PLI. Frontiers in Neuroanatomy. 2015;**9**:118. DOI: 10.3389/fnana.2015.00118

[4] Zilles K, Palomero-Gallagher N, Gräßel D, Schlömer P, Cremer M, Woods R, Amunts K, Axer M. High-resolution fiber and fiber tract imaging using polarized light microscopy in

the human, monkey, rat, and mouse brain. In: Rockland KS, editor. Axons and Brain Architecture. San Diego: Academic Press, Elsevier; 2016. pp. 369-389. DOI: 10.1016/B978-0-12-801393-9.00018-9

[5] Zeineh MM, Palomero-Gallagher N, Axer M, Gräßel D, Goubran M, Wree A, et al. Direct visualization and mapping of the spatial course of fiber tracts at microscopic resolution in the human hippocampus. Cerebral Cortex. 2017;**27**(3):1779-1794. DOI: 10.1093/cercor/bhw010

[6] Nieuwenhuys R. The myeloarchitectonic studies on the human cerebral cortex of the Vogt-Vogt school, and their significance for the interpretation of functional neuroimaging data. Brain Structure & Function. 2013;**218**:303-352. DOI: 10.1007/s00429-012-0460-z

[7] Axer M, Strohmer S, Gräßel D, Bücker O, Dohmen M, Reckfort J, Zilles K, Amunts K. Estimating fiber orientation distribution functions in 3D-polarized light imaging. Frontiers in Neuroanatomy. 2016;**10**:40

[8] Caspers S, Axer M, Caspers J, Jockwitz C, Jütten K, Reckfort J, et al. Target sites for transcallosal fibers in human visual cortex—A combined diffusion and polarized light imaging study. Cortex. 2015;**72**:40-53. DOI: 10.1016/j.cortex.2015.01.009

[9] Jones RC. A new calculus for the treatment of optical systems. Journal of the Optical Society of America. 1941;**31**:488-493

[10] Schober M, Schlömer P, Cremer M, Mohlberg H, Huynh AM, Schubert N, et al. Reference volume generation for subsequent 3D reconstruction of histological sections. In: Proceedings of Bildverarbeitung für die Medizin; Lübeck; 2015. pp. 143-148

[11] Papp EA, Leergaard TB, Calabrese E, et al. Waxholm space atlas of the Sprague Dawley rat brain. NeuroImage. 2014;**97**:374-386

[12] Schubert N, Axer M, Schober M, Huynh AM, Huysegoms M, Palomero-Gallagher N, Bjaalie JG, Leergaard TB, Kirlangic ME, Amunts K, Zilles K. 3D reconstructed cyto-, muscarinic M2 receptor, and fiber architecture of the rat brain registered to the Waxholm space atlas. Frontiers in Neuroanatomy. 2016;**10**:51

[13] Kjonigsen L, Lillehaug S, Bjaalie JG, et al. Waxholm space atlas of the rat brain hippocampal region: Three-dimensional delineations based on magnetic resonance and diffusion tensor imaging. NeuroImage. 2015;**108**:441-449

[14] Lorensen WE, Cline HE. Marching cubes: A high resolution 3D surface construction algorithm. In: Proc. of Computer Graphics and Interactive Techniques; 1987. pp. 163-169

[15] Levoy M. Display of surfaces from volume data. IEEE Computer Graphics and Applications. 1988;**8**(3):29-37

[16] Telea AC. Data Visualization: Principles and Practice. Boca Raton, FL, USA: CRC Press; 2015

[17] Gouraud H. Continuous shading of curved surfaces. IEEE Transactions on Computers. 1971;**C-20**(6):623-629

[18] Schubert N, Gräßel D, Pietrzyk U, et al. Visualization of vector fields derived from 3D polarized light imaging. In: Proceedings of Bildverarbeitung für die Medizin; Berlin. 2016. pp. 176-181

[19] Hänel C, Demiralp AC, Axer M, Gräßel D, Hentschel B, Kuhlen TW. Interactive level-of-detail visualization of 3D-polarized light imaging data using spherical harmonics. In: Eurographics Conference on Visualization; 2017

[20] Mori S, Crain BJ, Chacko VP, van Zijl PC. Three-dimensional tracking of axonal projections in the brain by magnetic resonance imaging. Annals of Neurology. 1999;**45**:265-269

[21] Basser PJ, Pajevic S, Pierpaloi C, Duda J, Aldroubi A. In vivo fiber tractography using DT-MRI data. Magnetic Resonance in Medicine. 2000;**44**:625-632

[22] Behrens TE, Berg HJ, Jbabdi S, Rushworth MF, Woolrich MW. Probabilistic diffusion tractography with multiple fibre orientations: What can we gain? NeuroImage. 2007; **34**:144-155

[23] Paxinos G, Watson C. The Rat Brain in Stereotaxic Coordinates. 7th ed. San Diego, USA: Academic Press, Elsevier; 2013

Chapter 4

Detection of Brain Tumor in MRI Image through Fuzzy-Based Approach

Neha Mathur, Yogesh Kumar Meena,
Shruti Mathur and Divya Mathur

Additional information is available at the end of the chapter

http://dx.doi.org/10.5772/intechopen.71485

Abstract

The process of accurate detection of edges of MRI images of a brain is always a challenging but interesting problem. Accurate detection is very important and critical for the generation of correct diagnosis. The major problem that comes across while analyzing MRI images of a brain is inaccurate data. The process of segmentation of brain MRI image involves the problem of searching anatomical regions of interest, which can help radiologists to extract shapes, appearance, and other structural features for diagnosis of diseases or treatment evaluation. The brain image segmentation is composed of many stages. During the last few years, preprocessing algorithms, techniques, and operators have emerged as a powerful tool for efficient extraction of regions of interest, performing basic algebraic operations on images, enhancing specific image features, and reducing data on both resolution and brightness. Edge detection is one of the techniques of image segmentation. Here from image segmentation, tumor is located. Finally, we try to retrieve tumor from MRI image of a brain in the form of edge more accurately and efficiently, by enhancing the performance of diffe rent kinds of edge detectors using fuzzy approach.

Keywords: fuzzy inference system (FIS), magnetic resonance imaging (MRI), nuclear magnetic resonance (NMR)

1. Introduction

The tumor refers to as a swelling in any part of body, which creates a lump or mass in the body. The term "tumor" which literally means swelling, can be applied to any pathological process that produces a lump or mass in the body. Tumors are the major characteristic of neoplasm's [1]. Neoplasm is a group of diseases term usually used for cancers. Sometimes while performing image diagnosis, doctors get confused between the diseases caused due to tumor and diseases caused due to infections. Sometimes it may happen that body cell loses its capacity to react towards the normal physiological mechanisms. The physiological mechanisms help to control the growth of such tissue. Due to which tumor get into place. Neoplastic tissue originates from the body cells due to uncontrolled growth and further can be indicated by the term tumor. In brain, tumor can be found in places such as neurons, blood vessels, skull, lymphatic tissue, pituitary and pineal gland. Brain tumor can be classified on the basis of their level of growth and also on the basis of resemblance with their parent cell. Based on their growth tumor can be classified as: benign tumor and malignant tumor. Benign tumors grow slowly and also do not spread to adjacent tissues whereas malignant tumor grows rapidly and get spread to the adjacent tissues. Based on their resemblance tumor can be classified as: differentiated and undifferentiated. Tumors that are different from their parent cell type are known as differentiated tumors and thus have slow growing rate. Tumors that seem like their parent cell type are known as undifferentiated tumors and thus have high growing rate. While growing, cells of tumor are shed into the surrounding extra cellular space and into the lymphatic system and are trapped in lymph nodes, where they begin to grow, and producing lymph node metastases.

The visualization of tumor depends on the surrounding tissue properties. These properties are physical or metabolic which when different from the tumor helps in visualizing the tumor. Otherwise the tumor boundary will be either distinct or fuzzy. A tumor can be differentiated from the normal tissue with the help of its matrix. This matrix can be textured, homogeneous based on the tumor type. The visualization of tumor boundary greatly depends on the surrounding tissues.

2. Objective

In recent years, segmentation of Magnetic Resonance (MR) image is a good research field requires detection of edges of a tumor in the brain. The purpose of edge detection is to generate an edge map based on the distribution of the intensity discontinuity of the image. The methods used for MRI of a brain have many disadvantages such as the noise and intensity in homogeneities are the two factors from which thresholding-based segmentation method gets affected. The region growing base segmentation method has a demerit as it requires manual interaction which helps in obtaining the seed point and also its noise sensitive nature and dependency on homogeneity that makes it a bad choice for segmentation. Region splitting and merging method are subject to a restriction of segmenting only those body parts that have well-defined boundaries such as lungs or bony structures. In order to obtain training data in classifier method, it requires manual interaction which then restricts it. Since no new data is generated for iteration, thus the usage of same data each time lead to unfair results which then cannot be used for differentiating between anatomical and physiological subjects related information. In order to choose an appropriate parameter that helps in placing an initial model, the boundary-based methods require manual interaction and are also more computationally expensive. Hybrid methods are insufficient for the segmentation of complex medical images. So, to make hybrid methods efficient enough to produce successful segmentation they are combined with powerful initialization techniques. In order to overcome the mentioned shortcoming of the above methods used for segmentation of brain MR image, edge detection using fuzzy approach. On the basis of the intensity histogram of an image, this system divides an image into multiple groups. These groups are determined on the basis of threshold values of an input image such that each group will have a different threshold value. To cluster the pixels into groups we have used k-means clustering where the pixels are grouped on the basis of their intensities and different groups are represented as the interval defined by two consecutive strong valleys on the intensity histogram of the image. The fuzzy-based automatic thresholding technique with k-means clustering improves the edge image when it is used by the classical Sobel operator.

3. Overview of brain MRI image segmentation

The Brain MRI image segmentation is a technique which involves study of the brain tumors, which can be detected easily from brain MR image [7]. While detecting the tumor; it involves techniques that differentiate different tumor area from Magnetic Resonance (MR) images. Magnetic resonance imaging (MRI) is used for brain imaging and is a high-quality medical imaging. This technique is useful to see the level of detail in the human body. Many imaging methods are developed for the early detection of brain tumors and also for its diagnostics purpose. As compared to other imaging techniques such as Positron Emission Tomography (PET), Magnetic Resonance Imaging (MRI), and Computed Tomography (CT), MRI is the most efficient one. These are the qualities of MRI, which make it efficient such as high contrast of soft tissues, high spatial resolution.

The important feature of MRI is that it does not produce any harmful radiation also it is reliable and has fast detection and classification of brain cancer. The brain tumor segmentation has many stages. When segmentation of brain MR images is done manually, the process gets time consuming and gets tedious. Thus to reduce manual interaction in brain MR image segmentation, there is a requirement of automatic methods.

3.1. Types of brain MRI image segmentation

The image processing techniques used for brain MRI image segmentation can be classified in three ways, the first way contains **region-based** methods, the second way contains **boundary-based** methods and the third way contains **hybrid** method. The following **Figure 1** represents the classification of brain image segmentation methods.

The segmentation methods which are used to segment a MRI image of a brain are as follows:

3.1.1. Region-based methods

Region is an important concept in the field of segmentation of an image. In an image of a scene a region may correspond as an object as pixels belonging to an object are grouped together and marked. The accurate segmentation of an image involves proper portioning of an image into different regions, which thus can be possible by using gray values of the pixels of an image. The region-based segmentation groups the pixels of an image, which are neighbors and also have similar values. The pixels having different values are split from each other.

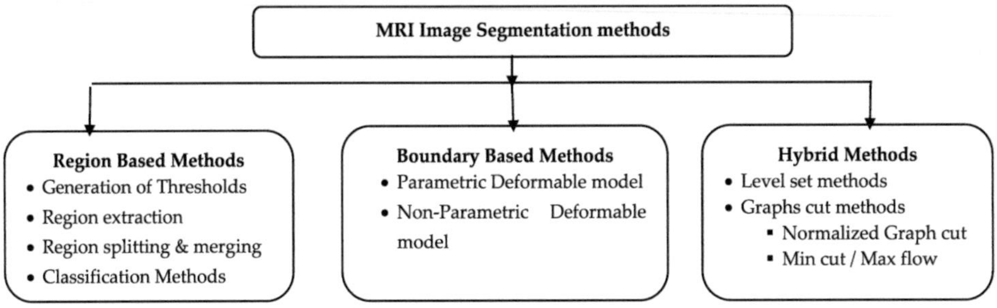

Figure 1. Block diagram of MRI image segmentation methods.

The region-based methods for segmentation of MRI image of a brain includes following approaches:

a. Generation of thresholds

In this technique images is assumed to be composed of different regions having different gray level ranges. Under the sequence of steps followed during image processing operations, thresholding is the initial step which is used to determine the intensity value of an image called the threshold, which generates the different classes. In this technique of segmentation the pixels are grouped according to the intensity between the two thresholds into one class. Thus, in this method more emphasis is given to the selection of good threshold. This approach-based methods generally deal with activities used to perform preprocessing of medical images and preregistration problems. But the spatial characteristics of an image are not considered by this method, which makes thresholding more sensitive to noise and intensity in homogeneity's, which occur in MRI images.

b. Region extraction

On the basis of some predefined criteria such as intensity information and edges in an image, etc. some regions of the image are being extracted. The first step of this technique requires an initial seed point which is useful in extracting regions connected to that seed point with same intensity value. The pixels or group of pixels belonging to the region of interest is known as seeds. In the second step, on the basis of homogeneous pixels in small neighboring regions are examined and selected pixels are added to the growing region. The above step repeats until and unless no more pixels are added to the growing region. Finally the object is detected from all the pixels that are added to the growing region. But this method has disadvantages that for extraction of each region of interest seed point is to be planted which requires manual interaction. Another demerit of region growing is that it is sensitive to noise and also its dependency on homogeneity criteria may cause extraction of those regions which are not of interest.

c. Region splitting and merging

This approach is the special case of region growing method, such that after applying region growing method when homogeneity criteria is not satisfied by a region, then a splitting method is applied which splits the region into four subregions. The splitting method continues until all regions satisfy the homogeneity criteria. In the final step of this technique, a quad tree having each vertex with exactly four descendent is generated and the leaf vertices of the quad tree represent homogeneous regions. This technique performs quite well while segmenting organs that have well-defined boundaries, such as lungs or bony structures. The major problem with this approach is the boundary leakage. As this method is a hierarchical approach to region-based image segmentation, so it also has the same disadvantage as the region growing have.

d. Classification methods

With the help of image data having prior known labels, a feature space is derived from them, which is the range space for any function of the image. Thereafter, classification methods implement efficient strategies to partition a feature space. It is based on the pattern recognition techniques.

3.1.2. Boundary-based methods

In this method an image is viewed as a collection of various objects. Each object is assumed to be composed of many solid shapes, by making outlining on the surface of objects into solid shapes with the help of parabolic lines. The objects get separated from the background due to which it's become easier to get information from an image.

This type of approach consists of the following method:

a. Parametric deformable model

Under the influence of internal and external forces, some curves or surfaces, gets deformed, the selection of these curves or surfaces is made by the parametric deformable model. In the MRI image when a tumor is present at the boundary of an object, it is extracted by placing a closed curve or surface near the desired boundary and then makes this as an input for an iterative relaxation process. The major disadvantage of this method is that for the selection of initial model and appropriate parameters, this method require manual interaction.

b. Non-parametric deformable model

Curve convolution theory and level set methods are the concepts on which this model is based on. There is no dependency on parameters for the evolution of the curve, but this involves expensive computations.

3.1.3. Hybrid methods

The hybrid method is the combination of above approaches containing advantages of above approaches. In this approach limits of interested region is determined with the help of segmentation of an image is achieved. In order to select threshold values several diffe rent methods exist which includes manual selection of thres hold value or an automatic computation of threshold value known as automatic thresholding [8–12]. This type of approach consists of the following methods:

a. Level set methods

To handle any of the cracks, concavities, convolution, splitting, or merging without the need of training data, level set methods are used [7]. But limitation of this method is the requirement of specifying initial curves and also good results will be provided only if these curves are placed in the symmetric form with respect to the object boundary. In order to produce successful segmentation complex medical images, Level set segmentation need to be combined with powerful initialization techniques.

b. Graph cut method

The concept of graph partitioning is used by this method under which each image is treated as a graph G such that the vertices of graph G are composed of pixels and in order to achieve image segmentation, weight of each edge is determined based on the vertices it relates.

The graph cut method can also be implemented using following methods:

i. Min-cut/max-flow method

Under this approach two reusable and non-overlapping search trees represented as tree S from sources and T from sink t are used. The direction of tree S is from parent node for children and the tree T has a direction from children to parent node. On the basis of outer border or inner border both tree either tree S or T can have active or passive nodes respectively. And those which are not present in either tree are known as free nodes. In some case min-cut algorithm for graph cuts can produce bad partition.

ii. Normalized graph cuts method

In this method measurement of dissimilarity among different groups and similarity within groups is computed. Using the above measure of similarity a MRI image of a brain gets segmented.

From the above content it is clear that, clustering methods are more suitable to implement for MRI image segmentation, but it needs some automation.

4. Overview of fuzzy logic

The Fuzzy logic is an approach in the field of computation which is rather than using usual "true or false" (1 or 0), which is used by modern computers as a Boolean logic, determines the "degrees of truth." Dr. Lotfi Zadeh from the University of California [2], at Berkeley in the 1960s, while working on the problem that how the computer can understand natural language, was the first one to present the idea of fuzzy logic. Natural language which is used for many activities in universe is not easily translated into the absolute terms of 0 and 1.

Fuzzy logic to some extent seems similar to the working of a human brain. A human brain while taking any decision or reaching to any result initially aggregates some related data, from that data generates some partial truths. These partial truths are further aggregated by human to create some new truths of higher level, when these truths exceed some threshold values, a decision is taken or certain resultant state is being reached e.g. motor reaction. The working of an artificial computer neural network and the expert systems is analogous to the above process.

The mathematical models are used in the classical control theory, required for the description of physical plant under idea but the core of fuzzy logic emphasis on the creation of a model made of human expert, who does not thinks in terms of mathematical models to control the plant [3].

Fuzzy systems have its application in following situations:

- Fuzzy system is used in situations where actions of a system are not well understood e.g. highly complex systems, and
- Another type of situation in which Fuzzy system is used is those situations whose solutions exist, but the solutions that exist are an approximate one.

Fuzzy logic was first utilized for practical applications by the Japanese in their high-speed Sendai train. With the help of fuzzy logic, Japanese was able to improve economy, comfort, and precision of the ride on the train [4].

Fuzzy logic has its applications in many areas such as: in Sony pocket computers for the recognition of hand written symbols; in helicopters for flight aid; In subway systems controlling to improve the driving comfort, precision of the halting, and power economy; in automobiles to improve fuel consumption; in washing machines controlling through single-button, in vacuum cleaners to provide automatic control to motor with recognition of surface condition and degree of soiling; and prediction systems for early recognition of earthquakes through the Institute of Seismology Bureau of Metrology, Japan [5].

5. Overview of fuzzy inference system

The mapping from a given input to an output is expressed by the fuzzy inference system using fuzzy logics. The resultant output helps in taking the decisions and detection of various patterns. The fuzzy inference system involves concept which is described in membership functions, logical operations, and if-then rules [2]. The fuzzy inference systems have application in the area such as automatic control, the data classification, decision analysis, expert systems, and the computer vision. Because of the multidisciplinary nature, the fuzzy inference systems can also be called as, fuzzy-rule-based systems, the fuzzy expert systems, the fuzzy modeling. A fuzzy inference process whose initial state starts from fuzzification and end at a state defuzzification is displayed by following **Figure 2**:

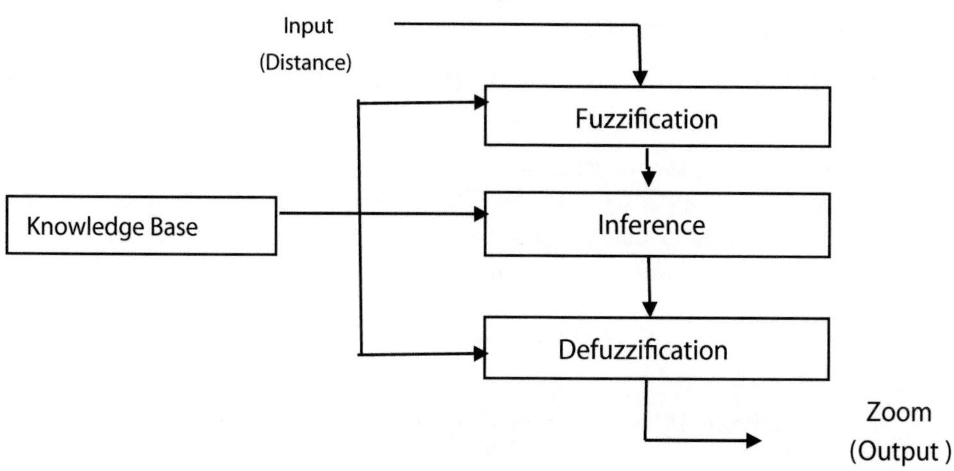

Figure 2. Fuzzy inference system.

The **Figure 2** above represents the Fuzzy inference process which comprises of five operations:

- Initially input variables get fuzzified.
- Then the fuzzy operator (AND or OR) are used in the antecedent.
- Implication from antecedent to the consequent.
- Aggregation of the consequents across rules.
- Defuzzification.

Sugeno-type fuzzy inference system was introduced in 1985 by Takagi-Sugeno-Kang [6] is similar to mamadanitype in the context of fuzzification and application of fuzzy operator. But sugeno type system has ouput membership functions either linear or constant.

6. Tumor detection using fuzzy-based K-means clustering system

The K-means segmentation method is used for further segmentation. In this method the procedure defines to obtain different threshold values, the histogram was segmented into groups/classes. Then this algorithm is used to calculate total image cluster centers, used to evaluate the most significant value of threshold. This proposed method is basically a measure of class separation. The local threshold method is used to find K-means segmentation threshold.

The basic steps of the algorithm of the proposed technique are:

i. Read the input MRI image 7.tif represented as $f(x, y)$.

ii. The histogram H of an input MRI image is generated. The histogram H is segmented using K-means segmentation method and gets divided into different groups (set of pixels). The groups generated for 7.tif MRI image are (0, 63), (64,137), (138,199), (200,255). The following **Figure 3** shows groups marked as the red circle on peak valleys, obtained after the segmentation of histogram H.

iii. An input MRI image $f(x, y)$ is convolved with Sobel kernel to generate gradient image $f'(x, y)$.

iv. Using fuzzy reasoning process, the Mean of edge magnitude, Mode and pixel count for the each group: (0, 63), (64,137), (138,199), (200,255) are calculated individually. Mode referred as most repeated value. Pixel count determines the number of pixels in the groups. The following equations are used to compute mode and pixel count.

$$\text{Mode}[K] = \text{calmode (group k)}; \quad (1)$$

$$\text{Pixel count}[K] = \text{Sum of pixels (group k)/sum of pixels (b)}; \quad (2)$$

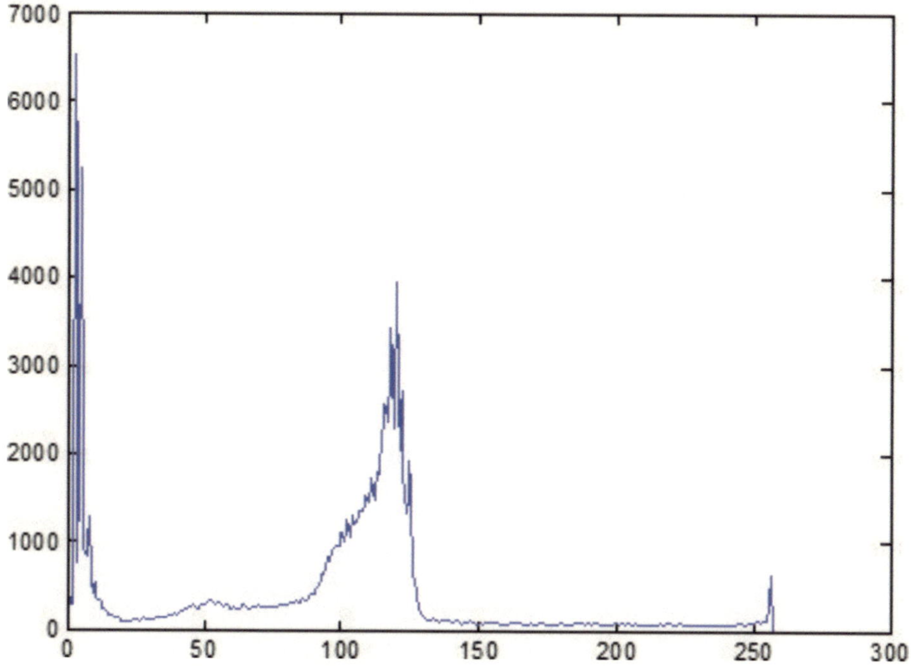

Figure 3. Image histogram after segmentation.

A mean of edge magnitude for a particular group is computed by using a mean value *mng*1 of pixels which is greater than group mean and a mean value *mng*2 of pixels which is lesser than group mean. Mean of edge magnitude for a particular group can be calculated using the below equation.

$$\text{Mean of the edge}[K] = |mng1 - mng2| \quad (3)$$

The parameters such as mean of an edge, mode and pixel count all are applied as an input to Fuzzy inference system whose membership functions for mode, mean edge, pixel count and output are represented in **Figures 4, 5, 6** and **7** respectively.

v. In this step each group is applied to the fuzzy inference system. Here group includes the parameters such as mean edge, mode and pixel count which are taken as an input values to be applied. Each system has its rule set, here in the proposed algorithm the fuzzy rule set for MIN-MAX Mamdani fuzzy inference system are used represented in the **Table 1**. The Fuzzy Inference System describes the rule base where 18 inference rules are determined. In the rule set three subsets are defined as "S" for small subsets, "M" for the medium subsets and "L" for large subsets. In the fuzzification process of fuzzy inference system these subsets are used to determine the effect of a particular group parameter. The output obtained from the fuzzy rule set is represented either in form of M or L. In the fuzzy rule set an output set is defined individually for each possible 18 combinations of S, M and L subsets for mean edge, mode and pixel count respectively for each group.

While working on the Mamdani fuzzy inference system there occur the following window shown in **Figure 8** which represents possible 18 combinations of S, M and L subsets for mean

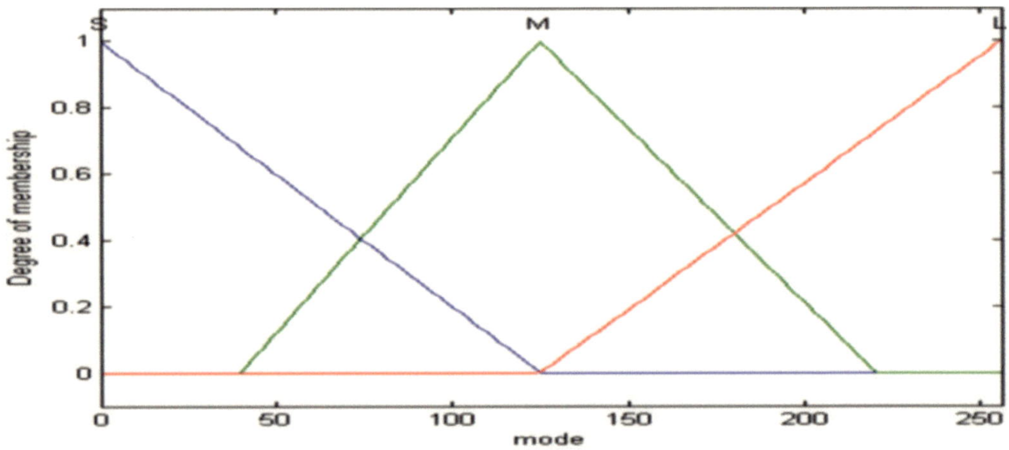

Figure 4. Membership function for mode.

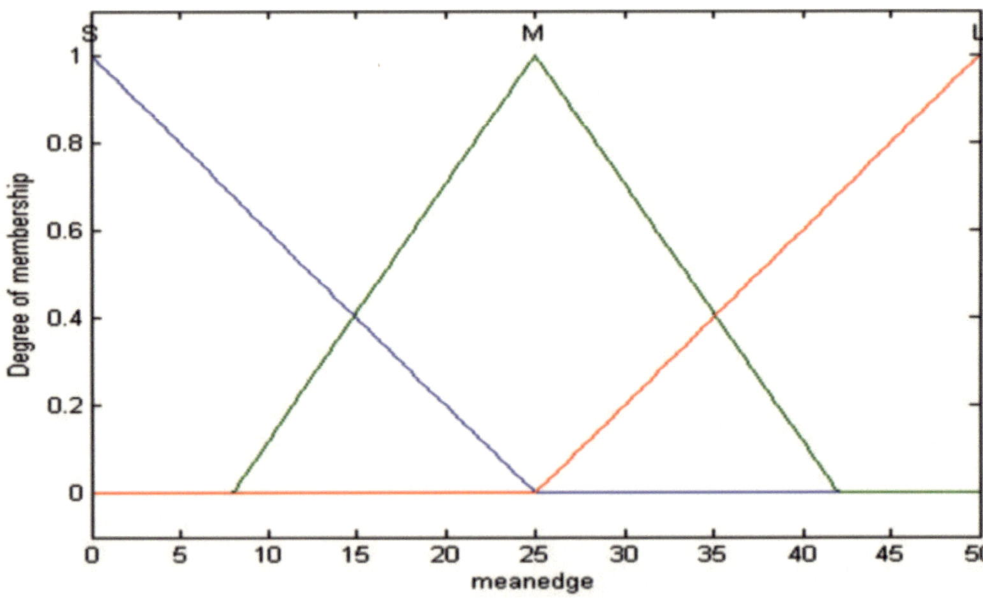

Figure 5. Membership function for mean edge.

http://dx.doi.org/10.5772/intechopen.71485

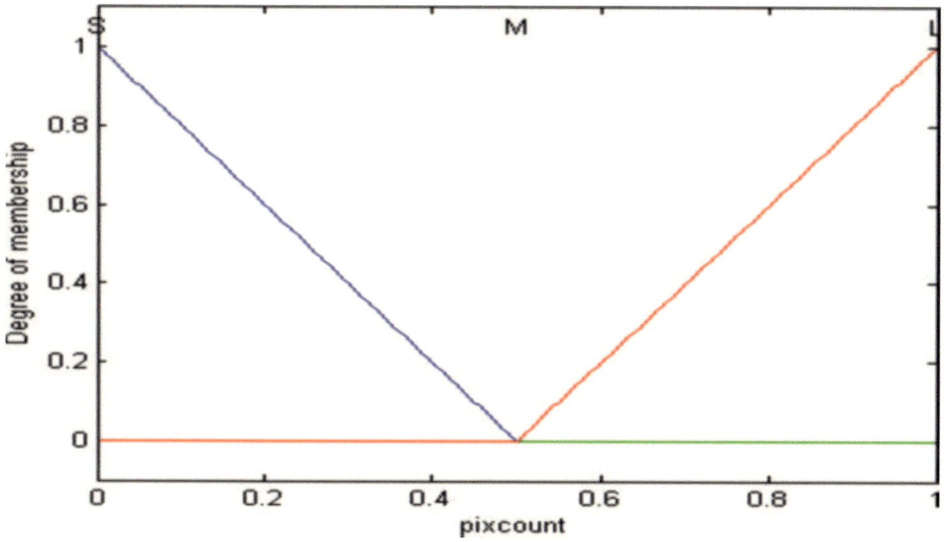

Figure 6. Membership function for pixel count.

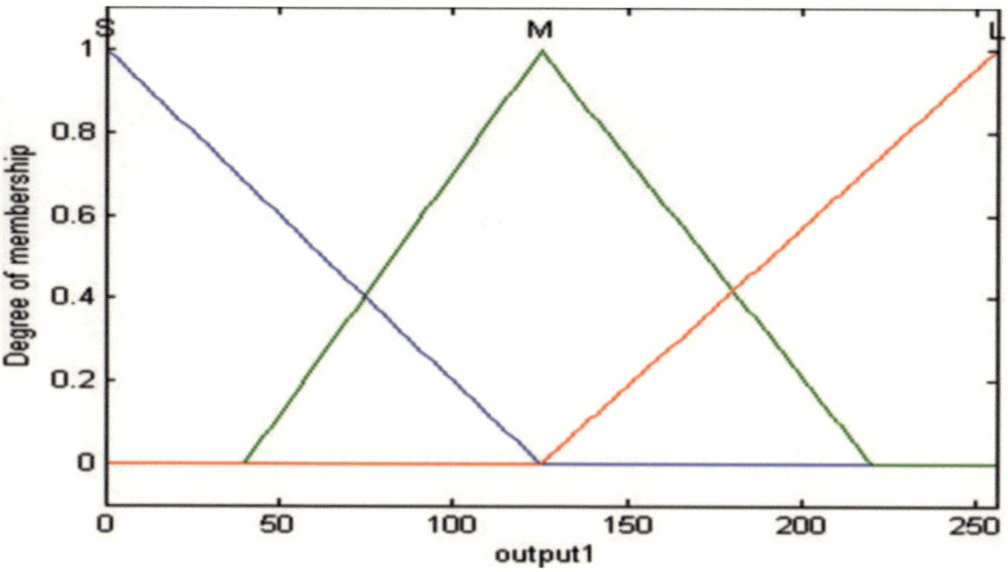

Figure 7. Membership function for output.

edge, mode and pixel count respectively for each group. The user can select the values of each subset on the basis of parameters of the group. Then on the basis of values of each subset, a particular output (either in form of M or L) will be generated.

Rules	1	2	3	4	5	6	7	8	9	10	11	12	13	14	15	16	17	18
Parameters																		
Mean edge	S	S	S	S	S	S	M	M	M	M	M	M	L	L	L	L	L	L
Mode	S	S	M	M	L	L	S	S	M	M	L	L	S	S	M	M	L	L
Pixel count	S	L	S	L	S	L	S	L	S	L	S	L	S	L	S	L	S	L
Output	M	M	M	M	M	M	M	M	M	L	M	L	M	L	M	L	L	L
Mean edge	S	S	S	S	S	S	M	M	M	M	M	M	L	L	L	L	L	L

Table 1. Fuzzy rules set for MIN-MAX Mamdani fuzzy inference system.

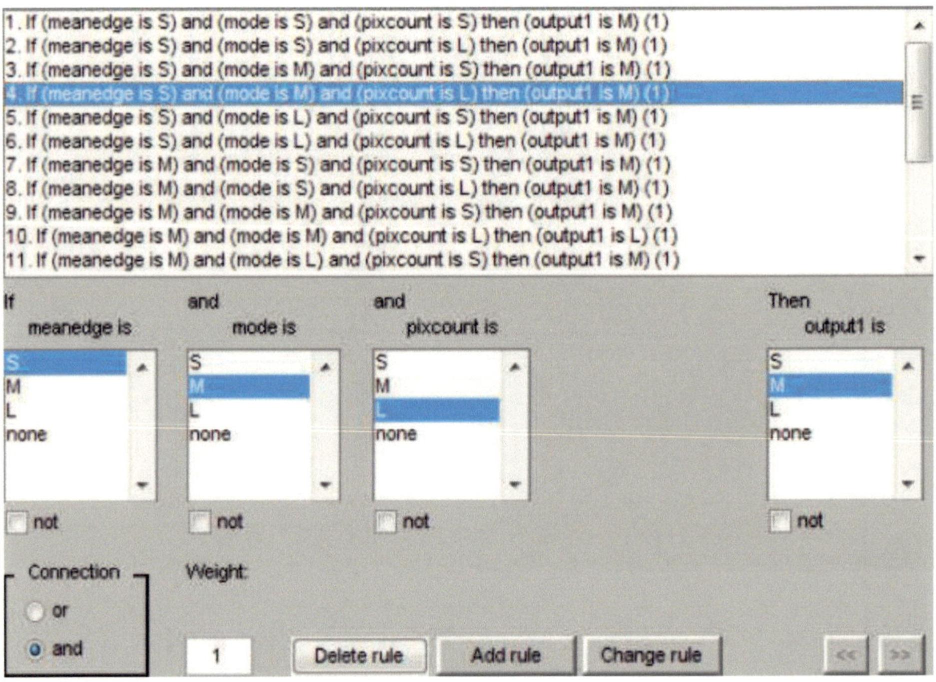

Figure 8. Selection of membership function through rule base.

vi. This step involves the process of defuzzification. The output value obtained above for each group is taken as an input to generate crisp scalar output value represented as $fuzzy_i$, for i^{th} group. The crisp scalar output value is used to determine threshold value for a particular group can be represented from the following equation:

$$t_i = mode_i + fuzzy_i \tag{4}$$

where t_i is the threshold value for the ith group, $mode_i$ is mode value of ith group, $fuzzy_i$ is output of fuzzy inference system defuzzification process for i^{th} group.

http://dx.doi.org/10.5772/intechopen.71485

S. No.	Input MRI image	Classical Sobel detection	Canny detection	Sobel detection with proposed method
1.	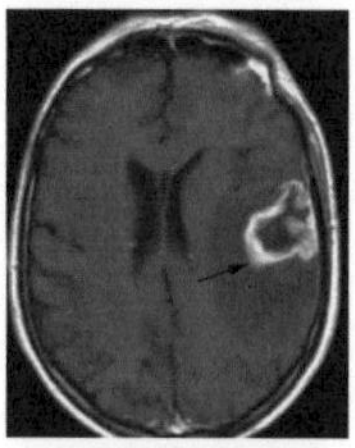	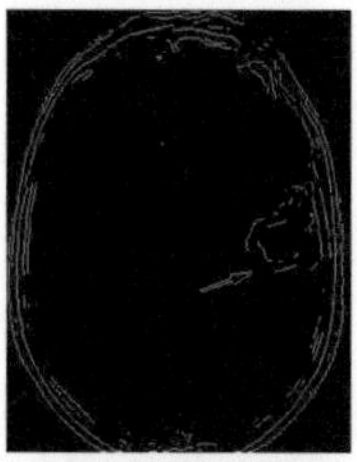	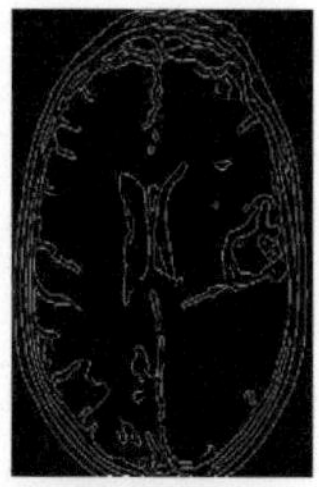	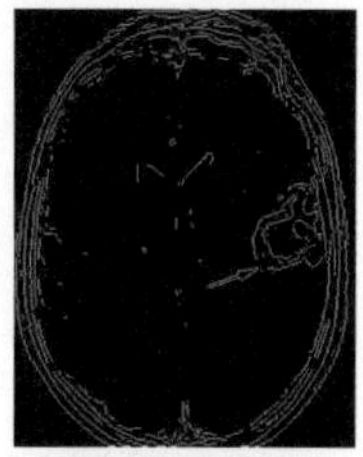
2.	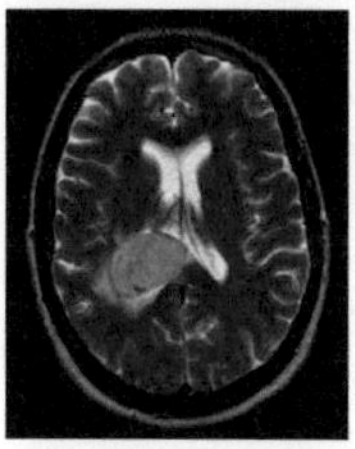	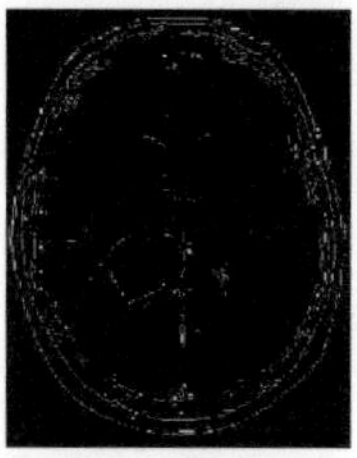	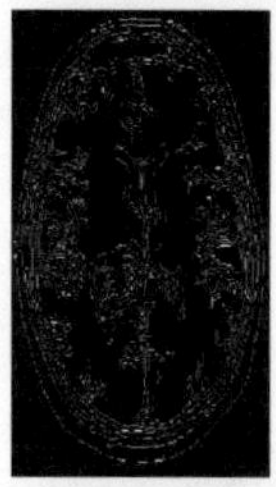	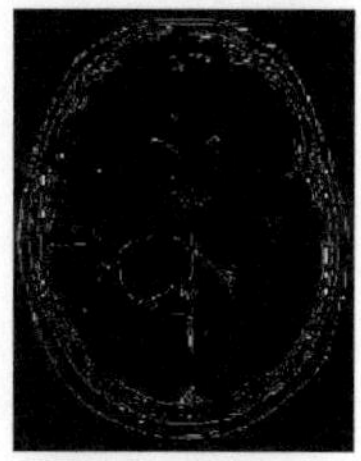
3.	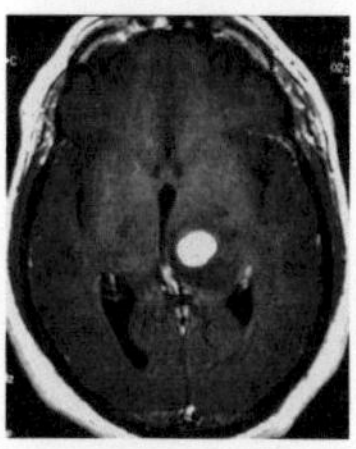	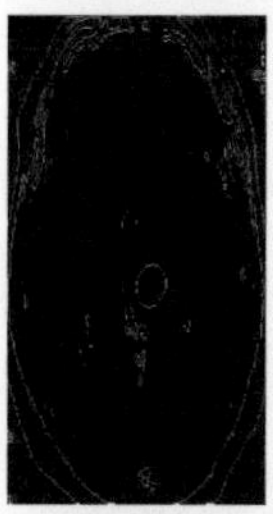	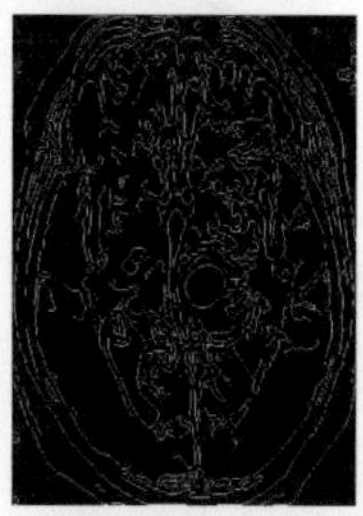	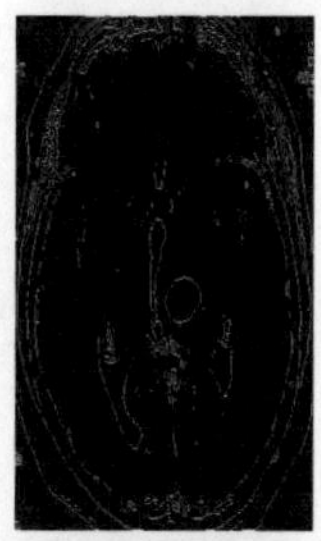
4.	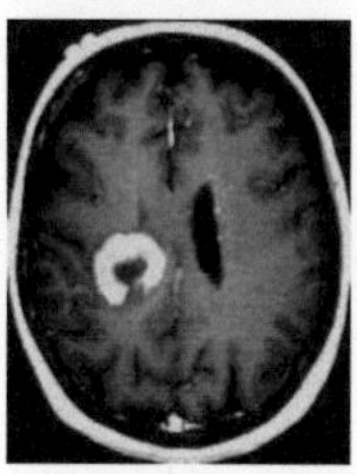	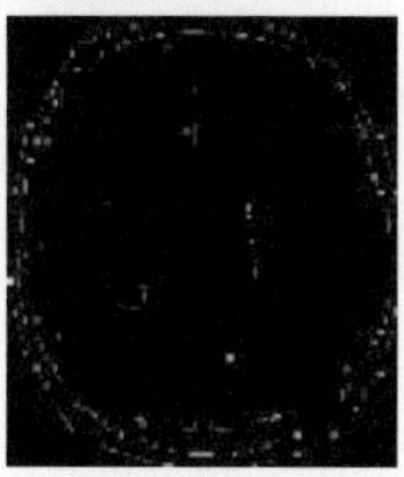	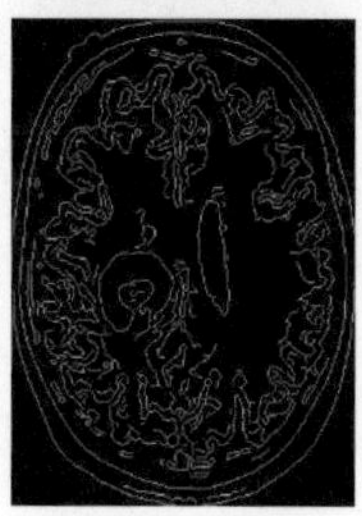	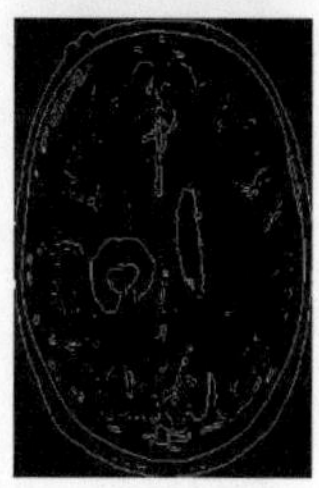

Table 2. Comparison of various edge detectors with proposed method.

vii. In the last step the final thresholds t_i for each group of histogram is applied independently to the gradient image $f'(x,y)$ generated in the third step. The output is an edge detected binary images shown in the last column of **Table 2**. The flow chart in **Figure 9** represents the basic steps of algorithm used for detection of edges in MRI image of a human brain. In the first step, the image is input into two systems: from the one system its histogram is generated and with the other system, known as Sobel edge kernel, image is convolved to generate a gradient image $f'(x, y)$. Then in the second step, different groups are generated from the histogram of an image by using k-means algorithm. These groups in the third step input into a fuzzy reasoning process used to compute the mean, mode and pixel

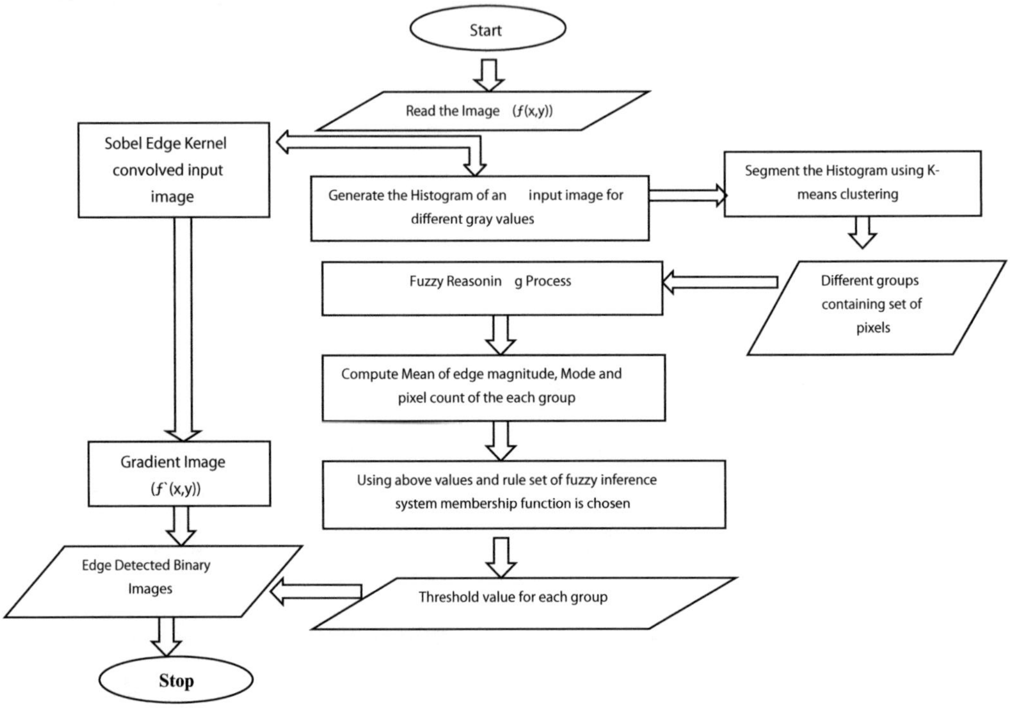

Figure 9. Flow chart showing steps of proposed approach.

count of each group. In the fourth step, membership function is computed for each group using above values of mean, mode and pixel count and rule set of Mamdani fuzzy inference system. In the last step, different threshold values are obtained. Then these threshold values and the gradient image $f'(x, y)$ is used to obtain final edge detected binary image.

7. Conclusion

In this method we take an MRI image of a human brain for edge detection. MRI image given as input to the system and its histogram segmented using our proposed method and get better results. In this step, a process must be executed after giving input, which checks all the required outputs and obtain the one which produces images in a proper and desired format. Each MRI image of a human brain is segmented while applying each type of edge detector. The performance evaluation of various edge detectors can be made by two ways. First on the basis of human judgment this is known as subjective method. Second on the basis of values of signal to noise ratio and mean square error between the edge detector image and the original image, this is known as an objective method. The edge detection is performed using automatic generation of threshold values using fuzzy approach. While using automatic thresholding approach the initial groups are computed using k-means clustering algorithm. Then for each obtained group a different threshold value is being generated using Mamdani fuzzy inference system rules set. These thresholds are then provided to Sobel edge detector. The comparison between the performance of edge detectors, by considering an edge detected image obtained by using edge detectors such as classical Sobel edge detector, canny edge detector and Sobel edge detector with proposed method is made on the basis of subjective method. The simulation results are shown in **Table 2**, whose first column represents the input of original MRI images 7.tif, 30.tif, 9.tif, 35.tif, respectively. The second, third and fourth column of table contains the output edge detected image obtained from the classical Sobel edge detector, Canny edge detector and modified Sobel edge detector using proposed method respectively.

In **Table 2**, the performance of classical Sobel and canny edge detectors on the basis of human judgment, compare with the performance of the improved Sobel edge detector implemented by the proposed method. After Serial number, the leftmost column shows the original image and the rightmost column shows the edge detected image of it obtained from the improved Sobel edge detector. The edge detected image obtained from the classical Sobel and canny edge detectors is presented by the second and third column respectively.

From the above result, it is clear that Canny edge detector provides over segmentation as it provides a large number of edges in an image which makes difficult to detect the tumor. Classical Sobel provides a limited number of edges, which in some images not even completes the boundary of tumor. When proposed method is applied to the classical Sobel, it enhances its performance by providing complete edges of the tumor.

Author details

Neha Mathur[1]*, Yogesh Kumar Meena[2], Shruti Mathur[3] and Divya Mathur[3]

*Address all correspondence to: nmdoll@gmail.com

1 Swami Keshvanand Institute of Technology Management and Gramothan, Jaipur, India

2 Malaviya National Institute of Technology, Jaipur, India

3 JECRC University, Jaipur, India

References

[1] Jain R, Kasturi R, Schunck BG. Machine Vision. McGraw-Hill, Inc.; 1995. pp. 140-185. ISBN 0-07-032018-7

[2] Zadeh L. Fuzzy sets. Information and Control. 1965;**353**:338-353

[3] Kerre EE, Nachtegal M. Fuzzy Techniques in Image Processing (Studies in Fuzziness and Soft Computing, 52). Physica Verlag; 2000

[4] Russo F. Edge detection in noisy images using fuzzy reasoning. IEEE Transactions on Instrumentation and Measurement. 1998;**47**(5):1102-1105

[5] CS Lee, Kuo Y-H. Adaptive fuzzy edge detection for image enhancement. Proceedings of IEEE World Congress on Computational Intelligence, vol. 2; May 1998. pp. 1542-1547, ISBN 0-7803-4863-X

[6] Tizhoosh HR. Fast Fuzzy Edge Detection. IEEE 0-7803-7461-4/02

[7] Balafar MA, Ramli AR, Saripan MI, Mashohor S. Review of brain MRI image segmentation methods. Artificial Intelligence Review, Springer Science. March 2010;**33**(3):261-274

[8] Pham DL, Xu CY, Prince JL. Current methods in medical image segmentation. Annual Review of Biomedical Engineering. August 2000;**2**:315-337, ISSN: 0269-2821

[9] Gonzalez RC, Woods RE, Eddins SL. Digital Image Processing Using MATLAB. New Delhi: Dorling Kindersley (India) Pvt. Ltd., McGraw-Hill; 2011, ISBN0071084789

[10] Shapiro LG, Stockman GC. Computer Vision. Prentice-Hall; 2001. pp. 279-325, ISBN 0130307963

[11] Mobahi H, Rao S, Yang A, Sastry S, Ma Y. Segmentation of natural images by texture and boundary compression. Proceedings of International Journal of Computer Vision (IJCV), Springer. October 2011;**95**(1):86-98, ISSN0920-5691

[12] Tang J, Peli E, Acton S. Image enhancement using a contrast measure in the compressed domain. IEEE Signal Processing Letters. October 2003;**10**(10):289-292, ISSN1070-9908

MRI RF-Induced Heating in Heterogeneous Human Body with Implantable Medical Device

Ran Guo, Jianfeng Zheng and Ji Chen

Additional information is available at the end of the chapter

http://dx.doi.org/10.5772/intechopen.71384

Abstract

Magnetic resonance imaging (MRI) radio frequency (RF)-induced heating is one of the most important concerns of MRI safety for patients, especially with orthopaedic healthcare products. In this chapter, numerical modelling and simulations were conducted to study the RF-induced heating within a 1.5T and 3T magnetic resonance (MR) environment. Numerical simulations were firstly conducted to study the difference between the cases of implantable medical devices inside the phantom and the human body. Then, numerical modelling were conducted to describe the difference of electromagnetic behaviours between the homogeneous phantom and heterogeneous human tissues. The MRI RF-induced heating due to an implantable medical device behaves significantly different in homogeneous media and in heterogeneous human body. For typical orthopaedic medical devices, such as healthcare products applied to shoulder, humerus, hip, femur and tibia, the properties of the RF-induced heating are different in general phantom and in human body. The hot spot location, as well as worst case configuration were evaluated and it was found that they were determined by the incident field and electromagnetic properties of medium. With further scaling, the RF-induced heating in human body for the orthopedic devices can be assessed by phantom studies.

Keywords: MRI, RF-induced heating, orthopedic implant, phantom

1. Introduction

Many of the MR-related injuries and the few fatalities that have occurred were the apparent result of failure to follow safety guidelines or of the use of inappropriate information related to the safety aspects of biomedical implants and devices [1–7]. The preservation of a safe MR environment requires constant attention to the care of patients and individuals with metallic implants and devices, because the variety and complexity of these objects constantly changes [5–7]. Therefore, to guard against accidents in the MR environment, it is important to understand the risk associated with implantable medical devices which may cause potential problems.

The radiofrequency coils could send energy, in the form of electromagnetic radiation, into the human body. Since the energy is in the radio frequency range, the radiation is not ionizing. But it still can influence biological tissue. During MR procedures, the majority of the RF power transmitted for imaging or spectroscopy (especially for carbon decoupling) is transformed into heat within the patient's tissue as a result of resistive losses, through convection, conduction, radiation or evaporation [8–18]. Thus, a potential concern in MRI is the heating of the body during image acquisition.

To evaluate the RF-induced heating, the specific absorption rate (SAR) is applied to determine how much electromagnetic energy is absorbed by the body. SAR is typically expressed in unites of watts per kilogram, or W/kg. So the SAR could be defined as:

$$SAR(r) = \frac{\sigma}{2\rho} E^2(r) \quad (1)$$

where E is the total electric field and σ and ρ are the conductivity and density of biological tissue, respectively. The temperature rise in human body or phantom could be calculated by the total SAR according to the bio heat equation. SAR depends on the pulse sequence and the size, geometry, and conductivity of the absorbing object. To ensure participant safety, SAR in MRI studies is limited to minimize temperature increases.

The first study of human thermal responses to RF radiation-induced heating during an MR procedure was conducted by Schaefer et al. [19]. Temperature changes and other physiological parameters were assessed in volunteer subjects exposed to relatively high, whole-body averaged SARs (approximately 4.0 W/kg). The data indicated that there were no excessive temperature elevations or other deleterious physiological consequences related to the exposure to RF radiation [19].

However, for patients with medical implants, MRI-related RF induced heating is potentially problematic. The evaluation of heating for an implant or device is particularly challenging because of the many factors that affect temperature increase in these items. Variables that impact heating include the following: the specific type of implant or device; the electrical characteristic of the implant or device; the RF wavelength of the MR system; the type of transmit RF coil that is used (i.e., transmit head versus transmit body RF coil); the amount of RF energy delivered (i.e., the specific absorption rate, SAR); the landmark position or body part undergoing MRI relative to the transmit RF coil; and the orientation or configuration of the implant or device relative to the source of transmit RF coil.

In this chapter, it shows the importance of evaluation the MRI-related RF induced heating issues for patient with implantable medical devices. Generally, the estimation and measurement is based on *in-vitro* numerical simulation and experiment. And assessment methods could be separated into active and passive medical implants, respectively, due to the configuration difference of these devices. With the help of the *in-vitro* evaluation methods, it provides a highly possible way to estimate the temperature increase for patient with implants or devices during MRI examination.

2. *In-vivo* and *in-vitro*

MRI may be contraindicated for a given patient primarily due to its potential risks associated with a metallic implant or device. Although many investigations have been performed using laboratory animals to determine thermoregulatory reactions to tissue heating associated with exposure to RF radiation, these experiments do not directly apply to the conditions that occur during MR procedures, nor can they be extrapolated to provide useful information for various reasons [20, 21]. For example, the pattern of RF absorption or the coupling of radiation to biological tissues is primarily dependent on the organism's size, anatomical features, duration of exposure, sensitivity of the involved tissues (e.g., some tissues are more "thermal sensitive" than others), and a myriad of other variables [14, 21, 22]. Furthermore, there is no laboratory animal that sufficiently mimics or simulates the thermoregulatory responses of an organism with the dimensions and specific responses to that of a human subject. Therefore, experimental results obtained in laboratory animals cannot be simply "scaled" or extrapolated to predict thermoregulatory or other physiological changes in human subjects exposed to RF radiation-induced heating during MR procedures [14, 15, 22], and. In consideration of the above, *in-vitro* testing is performed to assess the various MRI issues for implants and devices in order to properly characterize the possible risks.

One of *in-vitro* methods is to use standard American Society for Testing and Materials (ASTM) phantom. ASTM F2182-11A depicts the guideline to measure the RF heating induced by implanted medical devices in a standard phantom filled with gelled-saline which mimic the muscles [23]. Studies have been conducted to evaluate the RF heating induced by orthopedic implants. Commonly a phantom or homogenous media is used to mimic the environments as the implants locate in human body in experiments and/or numerical simulations [24–32].

Although the RF-induced heating evaluating method using the phantom filled with gelled-saline is widely used, it is obvious that the RF environment of a human body and a phantom filled with gelled-saline are quite different. The power deposition due to an implant for a given incident RF field is a function of the physical properties of the implant and electrical properties of the surrounding medium. Compared with homogeneous gelled-saline in phantom, human body is an inhomogeneous circumstance which includes different tissues with various permittivity and conductivity in a wide range. Hence, it is necessary to study a feasible guide with *in-vitro* phantom to assess the RF-induced heating in heterogeneous human body.

2.1. Human body: heterogeneous medium

With the development of computational electromagnetics, anatomical computer models of the human body have been used for nearly four decades for dosimetric applications in electromagnetics (EM) [33] and in medical radiation physics [34]. The most prominent numerical

Name	Age (years)	Gender	Height (m)	Mass (kg)	BMI (kg/m²)
Duke	34	Male	1.74	70	23.1

Table 1. The characteristics of the anatomical Duke model.

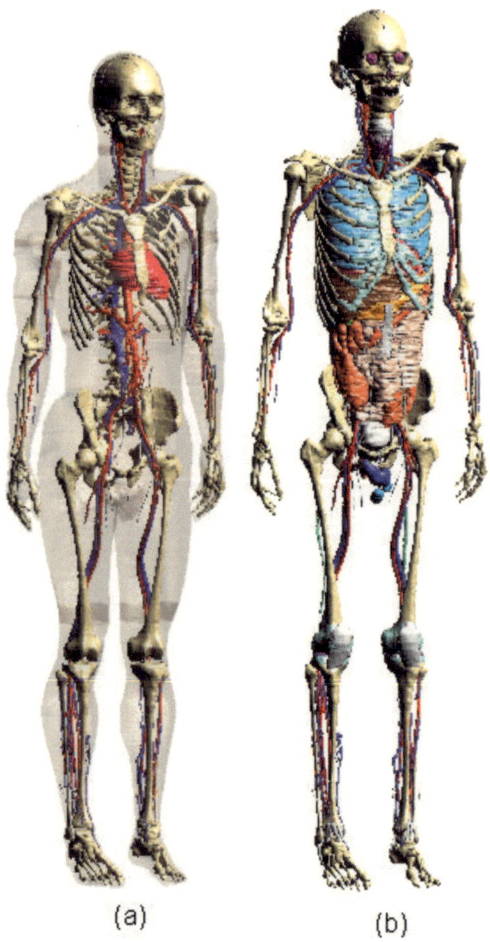

Figure 1. The segmented tissues and organs of anatomic body.

methods used in computational dosimetry of electromagnetic fields are based on finite-difference formulations of the underlying differential equations. For the simulation of both RF fields and induced tissue heating, the finite-difference time-domain (FDTD) method in its formulations by Yee [35] and Patankar [36] is applied to rectilinear grids to optimally handle large voxel models. The reconstructed human model used in this Chapter is from the Virtual Family [37]. It is based on high resolution magnetic resonance images of healthy volunteers. Seventy seven different tissue types were distinguished during the segmentation. Currently,

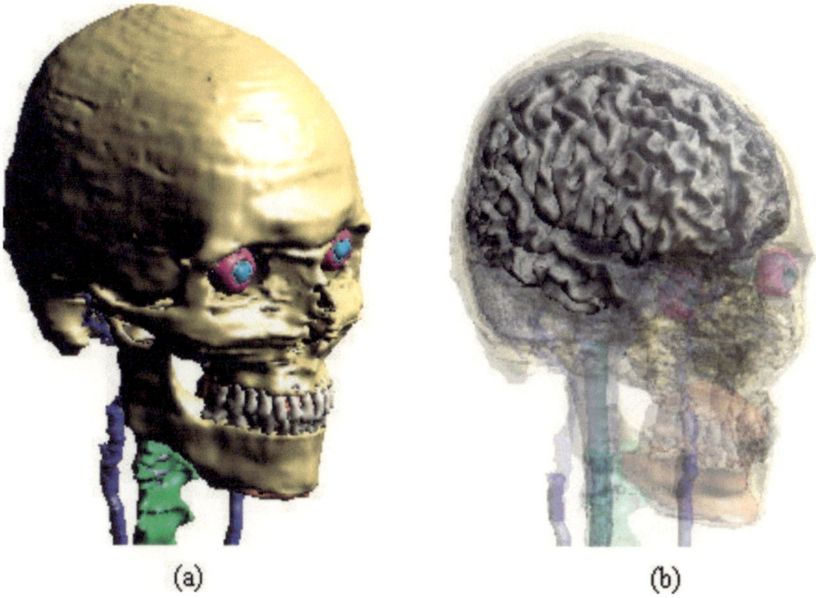

Figure 2. The segmented tissues and organs of anatomic brain.

Tissue or organ	Electric conductivity (S/m)		Relative permittivity		Density (kg/m³)
	1.5 T/64 MHz	3 T/128 MHz	1.5 T/64 MHz	3 T/128 MHz	
Adrenal gland	0.778305	0.804166	73.9472	66.7839	1027.5
Air internal	0	0	1	1	1.2
Artery	1.20667	1.24863	86.4441	73.159	1049.75
Bladder	0.287352	0.298014	24.5943	21.8607	1035
Blood vessel	1.20667	1.24863	86.4441	73.159	1049.75
Bone	0.0595255	0.0673524	16.6812	14.7171	1908
Brain gray matter	0.510868	0.58673	97.4294	73.5204	1044.5
Brain white matter	0.291504	0.342151	67.8358	52.5338	1041
Bronchi	0.528415	0.559346	58.8896	50.5714	1101.5
Bronchi lumen	0	0	1	1	1.2
Cartilage	0.452103	0.488375	62.9145	52.9242	1099.5
Cerebellum	0.719003	0.829397	116.35	79.7377	1045
Cerebrospinal fluid	2.06597	2.14301	97.3124	84.0406	1007
Commissure anterior	0.291504	0.342151	67.8358	52.5338	1041
Commissure posterior	0.291504	0.342151	67.8358	52.5338	1041
Connective tissue	0.474331	0.498727	59.4892	51.8568	1525
Cornea	1.00058	1.05874	87.3779	71.4566	1050.5

Tissue or organ	Electric conductivity (S/m)		Relative permittivity		Density (kg/m³)
	1.5 T/64 MHz	3 T/128 MHz	1.5 T/64 MHz	3 T/128 MHz	
Diaphragm	0.688213	0.719235	72.2347	63.4948	1090.4
Ear cartilage	0.452103	0.488375	62.9145	52.9242	1099.5
Ear skin	0.43575	0.522704	92.1679	65.437	1109
Epididymis	0.884871	0.926404	84.5272	72.1279	1082
Esophagus	0.877842	0.912807	85.8204	74.895	1040
Esophagus lumen	0	0	1	1	1.2
Eye lens	0.28588	0.312684	50.3392	42.7911	1075.5
Eye sclera	0.882673	0.917665	75.2998	64.9991	1032
Eye vitreous humor	1.50315	1.50536	69.1264	69.0619	1004.5
Fat	0.0661558	0.0697299	13.6436	12.3711	911
Gall bladder	1.48179	1.5764	105.443	88.8995	928
Heart lumen	1.20667	1.24863	86.4441	73.159	1049.75
Heart muscle	0.678423	0.766108	106.514	84.2573	1080.8
Hippocampus	0.510868	0.58673	97.4294	73.5204	1044.5
Hypophysis	0.778305	0.804166	73.9472	66.7839	1053
Hypothalamus	0.778305	0.804166	73.9472	66.7839	1053
Intervertebral disc	0.452103	0.488375	62.9145	52.9242	1099.5
Kidney cortex	0.741316	0.852313	118.556	89.6168	1049
Kidney medulla	0.741316	0.852313	118.556	89.6168	1044
Large intestine	0.638152	0.705214	94.6639	76.5722	1088
Large intestine lumen	0.688213	0.719235	72.2347	63.4948	1045.2
Larynx	0.452103	0.488375	62.9145	52.9242	1099.5
Liver	0.447984	0.510897	80.5595	64.2507	1078.75
Lung	0.288977	0.315616	37.1022	29.4677	394
Mandible	0.0595255	0.0673524	16.6812	14.7171	1908
Marrow	0.154335	0.162021	16.4355	13.5377	1028.5
Medulla oblongata	0.719003	0.829397	116.35	79.7377	1045.5
Meniscus	0.452103	0.488375	62.9145	52.9242	1099.5
Midbrain	0.719003	0.829397	116.35	79.7377	1045.5
Mucosa	0.488039	0.544202	76.7233	61.5852	1102
Muscle	0.688213	0.719235	72.2347	63.4948	1090.4
Nerve	0.312174	0.353802	55.0621	44.0653	1075
Pancreas	0.778305	0.804166	73.9472	66.7839	1086.5
Patella	0.0595255	0.0673524	16.6812	14.7171	1908

Tissue or organ	Electric conductivity (S/m)		Relative permittivity		Density (kg/m^3)
	1.5 T/64 MHz	3 T/128 MHz	1.5 T/64 MHz	3 T/128 MHz	
Penis	0.429311	0.478934	68.6368	55.9888	1101.5
Pharynx	0	0	1	1	1.2
Pineal body	0.778305	0.804166	73.9472	66.7839	1053
Pons	0.719003	0.829397	116.35	79.7377	1045.5
Prostate	0.884871	0.926404	84.5272	72.1279	1045
SAT	0.0661558	0.0697299	13.6436	12.3711	911
Skin	0.43575	0.522704	92.1679	65.437	1109
Skull	0.0595255	0.0673524	16.6812	14.7171	1908
Small intestine	1.59145	1.69285	118.363	87.9725	1030
Small intestine lumen	0.688213	0.719235	72.2347	63.4948	1045.2
Spinal cord	0.312174	0.353802	55.0621	44.0653	1075
Spleen	0.743914	0.835186	110.559	82.8917	1089
Stomach	0.877842	0.912807	85.8204	74.895	1088
Stomach lumen	0.688213	0.719235	72.2347	63.4948	1045.2
Teeth	0.0595255	0.0673524	16.6812	14.7171	2180
Tendon ligament	0.474331	0.498727	59.4892	51.8568	1142
Testis	0.884871	0.926404	84.5272	72.1279	1082
Thalamus	0.510868	0.58673	97.4294	73.5204	1044.5
Thymus	0.778305	0.804166	73.9472	66.7839	1023
Thyroid gland	0.778305	0.804166	73.9472	66.7839	1050
Tongue	0.652145	0.687137	75.2998	64.9991	1090.4
Trachea	0.528415	0.559346	58.8896	50.5714	1080
Trachea lumen	0	0	1	1	1.2
Ureter Urethra	0.429311	0.478934	68.6368	55.9888	1101.5
Vein	1.20667	1.24863	86.4441	73.159	1049.75
Vertebrae	0.0595255	0.0673524	16.6812	14.7171	1908

Table 2. The electromagnetic properties of the segmented tissues and organs.

the models are being widely applied in several studies on electromagnetic exposure, device optimization and medical applications. **Table 1** shows the characteristics of the anatomical model. Duke model is an anatomical model of adult male which is shown in **Figures 1** and **2**. And **Table 2** shows the segmented tissues and organs of the model, as well as the electromagnetic properties.

2.2. ASTM phantom: *in-vitro* measurement

The standard F2182 describe a test method for measurement of RF induced heating on or near passive implants and its surrounding during MRI procedure. A design of phantom container is introduced in the standard with its dimension shown in **Figure 3**. The material of phantom container are electrical insulators and non-magnetic and non-metallic. The phantom container is filled with a gelled-saline which has a relative permittivity $\varepsilon_r = 80.4$ and conductivity of $\sigma = 0.47$ S/m. In order to have a great conductivity and viscosity, a suitable gelled saline should be made with 1.32 g/L NaCl and 10 g/L polyacrylic acid (PAA) in water. Numerical simulations indicate that the maximum electric field inside the ASTM phantom is at mid-axial plane about 2 cm away from the vertical phantom side wall. To maximize the heating, and thereby maximizing the signal-to-noise ratio, we placed the implants at this location.

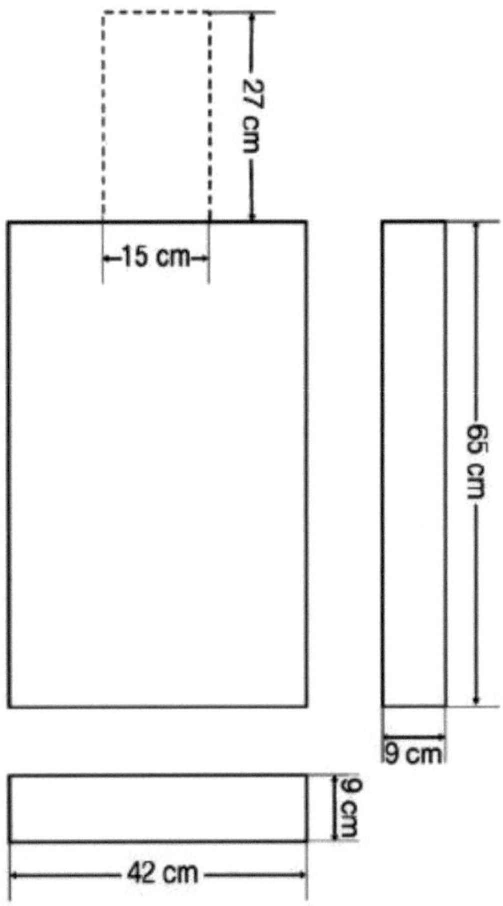

Figure 3. The structure and dimension of standard ASTM phantom.

http://dx.doi.org/10.5772/intechopen.71384

A generic RF transmit body coil is developed and shown in **Figure 4**. The upper plots represent a 1.5 T RF coil and the lower two plots represent a 3 T RF coil. A physical coil is usually difficult to model and it takes much longer simulation time to reach the steady state of the simulation. It has been shown that using a non-physical coil could significantly reduce the simulation time while providing the same result as that from a physical coil. Thus, rather than modeling the exact physical coil, the non-physical coils were modeled in this study. The two coils have the same dimensions, and both have 8 rungs. The diameter of the RF coil is 63 cm, and the height of the RF coil is 65 cm. The eight parallel lines or the rungs are one dimensional line current excitation. The end rings on top and bottom of the RF coils are tuning capacitors which are also modelled as one dimensional line segments.

The capacitance value is determined from several broadband simulations so that the second highest resonant frequency was adjusted to 64 MHz for 1.5-T and 128 MHz for 3-T systems. The detailed steps are: set an initial capacitance value for all capacitors on end rings and add a broadband pulse signal on one single rung. The other seven rungs are modeled as zero ohm resistors. After the simulation is finished, the power spectrum is extracted. If the second highest resonant frequency is not at appropriate resonant frequencies, the capacitance needs to be adjusted. From this study, the capacitance for the end ring tuning capacitor values is 7.2 pF for 1.5-T RF coil and 1.3 pF for 3-T RF coil.

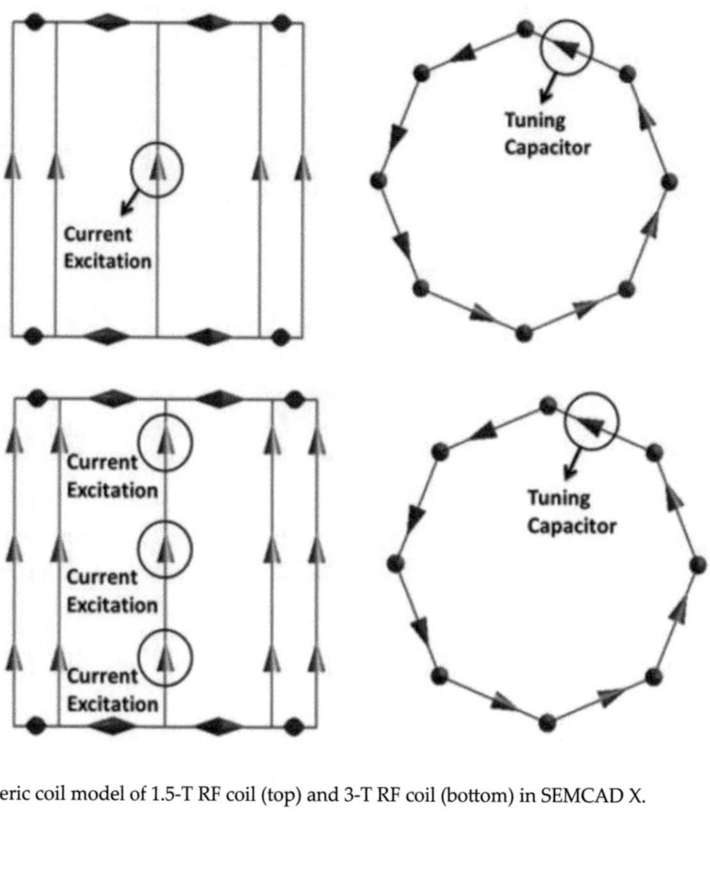

Figure 4. The generic coil model of 1.5-T RF coil (top) and 3-T RF coil (bottom) in SEMCAD X.

3. Passive implantable medical device

Any device intended to be totally or partially introduced into the human body through surgical intervention and intended to remain in place after the procedure for at a long-term duration is considered as an implantable device. Passive devices in terms of their form of operation can be classified as device used for transportation and storage of pharmaceutical liquid, device for alteration of blood, body fluids, medical dressing, surgical instruments; reusable surgical instruments, disposable aseptic device, implantable device, device for contraception and birth control, device for sterilization and cleaning, patient care device, in vitro diagnostic reagent, as well as other passive contacting device or passive supplementary device.

In this chapter, three typical categories of orthopedic implantable devices, bone plate system, hip prostheses and tibia intramedullary nails, are selected for MRI related RF induced heating study which are shown in **Figures 5–7**. The configuration of each implantable device is shown

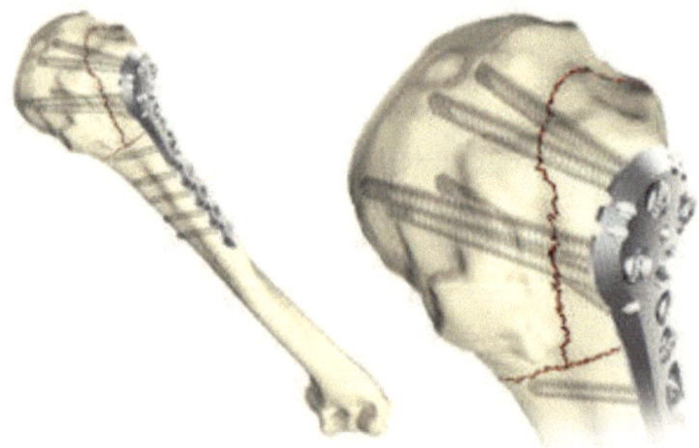

Figure 5. The bone plant system of AxSOS system from Stryker®.

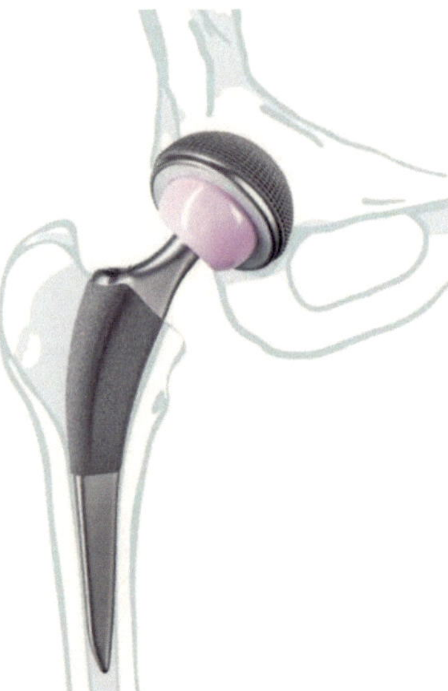

Figure 6. The hip prostheses of Excia® T from Aesculap®.

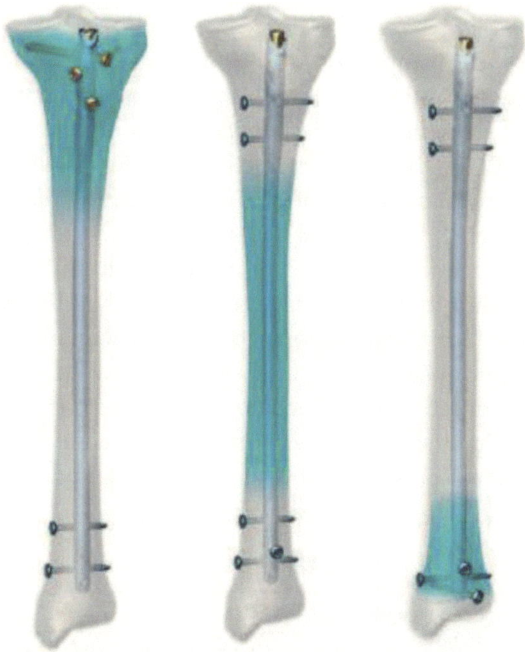

Figure 7. The tibia intramedullary nails of PROTect™ from Depuy Synthes.

in figure. For bone fragment compression plate, it is designed to offer multiple compression and reconstruction plating options for the treatment of bone fractures. The application of hip prostheses is related to hip revision and arthroplasty. As for intramedullary nails, they are characterized by the anatomic shape, which is intended to replicate the natural anatomic shape of the bones. They have been designed to help restore the shape of the bone and treat the fractured bones.

4. Numerically evaluate RF-induced heating

4.1. FDTD method

In this numerical investigation, we use the finite difference time domain (FDTD) based SEMCAD X 14.8 (SPEAG) simulation platform. Graphics processing unit (GPU) hardware acceleration was achieved using the SPEAG CUDA library with Tesla C2075 graphic card which is can handle up to 90 million cells. To assure convergence of the numerical simulations, the simulation time was set to 20 periods for each simulation. Additionally, the convergence was checked after the simulations were finished. The material of orthopedic devices is set to perfect electric conductor (PEC), and all the numerical results are normalized to a whole body average SAR of 2 W/kg. The SAR distribution is studied for each case.

4.2. Bone plate system

To ensure a comprehensive comparison, the 1g local average peak SAR value at device is extracted for each configuration of femur and humerus system. **Tables 3** and **4** show the value for femur and humerus system. For each numerical result, whole-body average SAR is normalized to 2 W/kg. Since the interaction between RF induced field and implant is dependent on the physical structure of device, the heating effect variations related to the length of plate and screw are studied separately. For femur system, the plate length varies from 100 to 300 mm, and the screw length changes from 10 to 32 mm. For humerus system, the screw dimension is the same as femur system. But the plate length varies only from 100 to 250 mm due to the limit of bone structure. The plate length is studied at first for minimum and maximum screw length. Then the screw length is investigated under the worst case of plate length study which has the highest 1g average peak SAR value for *in-vivo* simulation. **Figures 8–13** show the results which are corresponding to femur and humerus plate system. The solid and dash curve and indicate the *in-vivo* and *in-vitro* results, respectively.

Plate length (mm)		Screw length (mm)	1.5 T/64 MHz		3 T/128 MHz	
			In-vivo SAR_{1g} (W/kg)	*In-vitro* SAR_{1g} (W/kg)	*In-vivo* SAR_{1g} (W/kg)	*In-vitro* SAR_{1g} (W/kg)
100		10	64.20	125.97	79.75	80.90
150		10	94.82	178.62	74.52	64.01
175		10	107.00	190.44	68.50	50.20
200		10	116.65	188.87	63.37	44.69
225		10	117.00	185.04	63.10	37.72
250		10	123.00	169.75	61.23	37.27
275		10	117.00	149.81	53.80	35.33
300		10	105.00	134.91	42.37	38.53
100		32	85.02	100.22	88.26	71.90
150		32	108.17	135.90	55.48	47.74
200		32	104.91	140.27	51.56	41.59
250		32	111.73	123.17	48.94	37.09
300		32	79.94	128.93	27.77	40.70
250(1.5 T)	100(3 T)	15	120.00	150.91	79.30	72.19
250(1.5 T)	100(3 T)	20	121.00	135.71	76.20	68.00
250(1.5 T)	100(3 T)	25	123.00	132.15	64.2	66.52

Table 3. Peak 1g averaged SAR of femur system for *in-vivo* and *in-vitro* cases.

Plate length (mm)	Screw length (mm)	1.5 T/64 MHz		3 T/128 MHz	
		In-vivo SAR_{1g} (W/kg)	*In-vitro* SAR_{1g} (W/kg)	*In-vivo* SAR_{1g} (W/kg)	*In-vitro* SAR_{1g} (W/kg)
100	10	38.02	135.61	65.47	90.51
150	10	63.74	192.14	94.68	59.90
200	10	69.47	204.57	81.84	45.54
250	10	104.57	193.61	86.73	41.50
100	32	30.70	92.17	63.46	64.6
150	32	54.10	124.76	85.39	53.70
200	32	55.90	161.97	75.19	43.39
250	32	109.00	156.38	108.92	42.51
250	15	95.53	161.64	77.82	35.33
250	20	91.02	163.55	72.91	38.94
250	25	88.27	164.54	68.40	41.32

Table 4. The peak 1g average SAR value of humerus system for *in-vivo* and *in-vitro* cases.

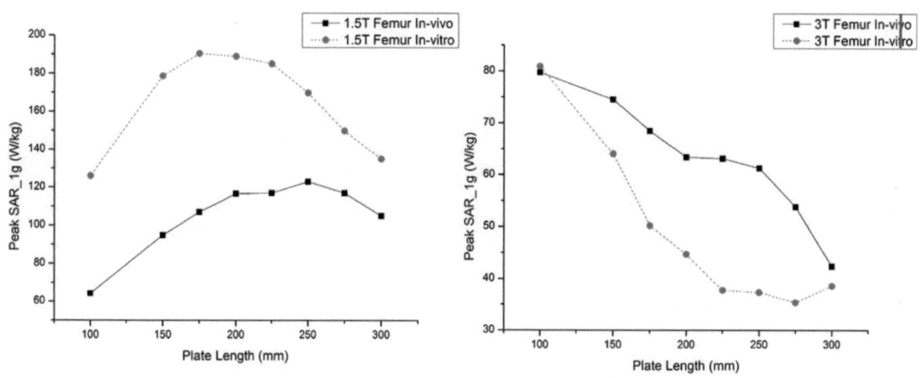

Figure 8. The femur bone plate length study of 10 mm screw for 1.5 T (left) and 3 T (right).

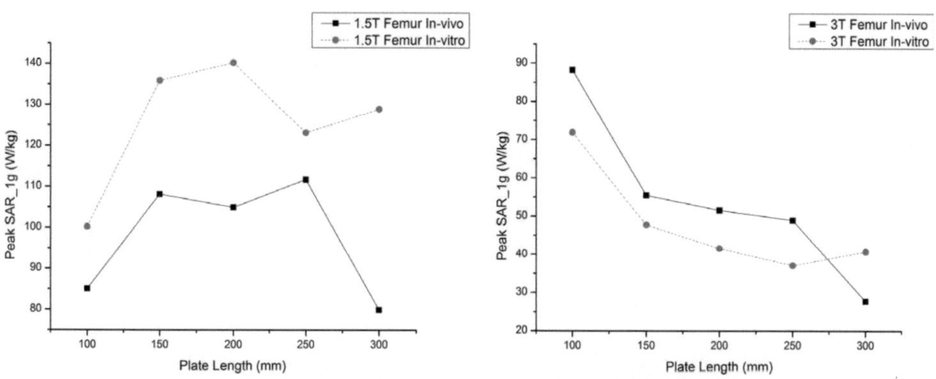

Figure 9. The femur bone plate length study of 32 mm screw for 1.5 T (left) and 3 T (right).

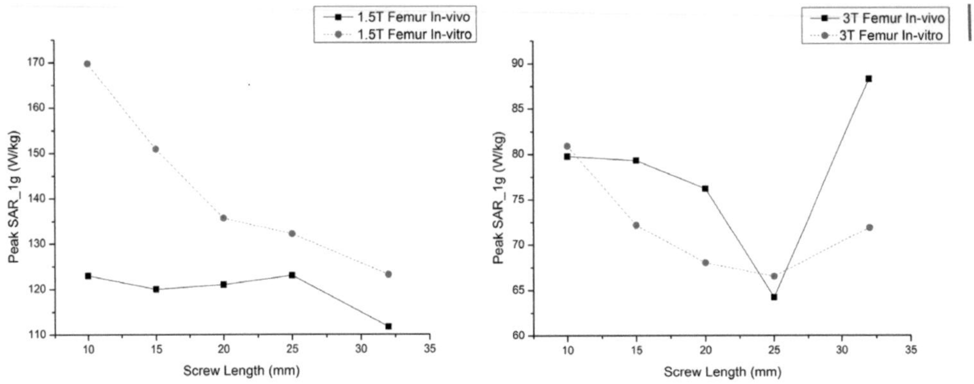

Figure 10. The femur screw length study for 1.5 T (left) and 3 T (right).

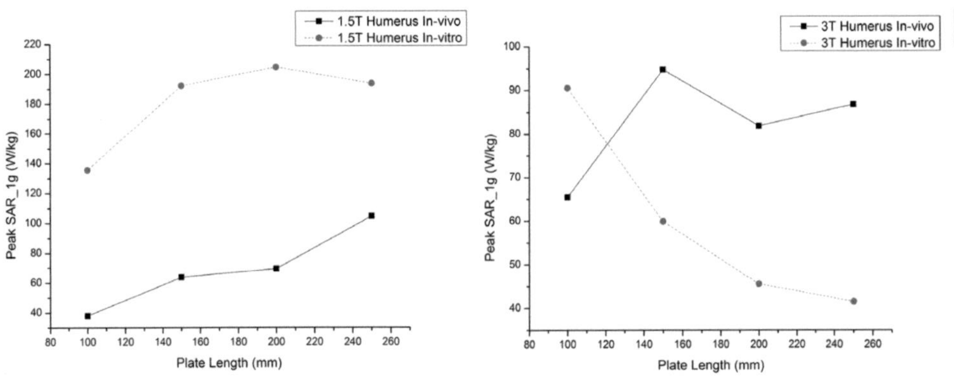

Figure 11. The humerus bone plate length study of 10 mm screw for 1.5 T (left) and 3 T (right).

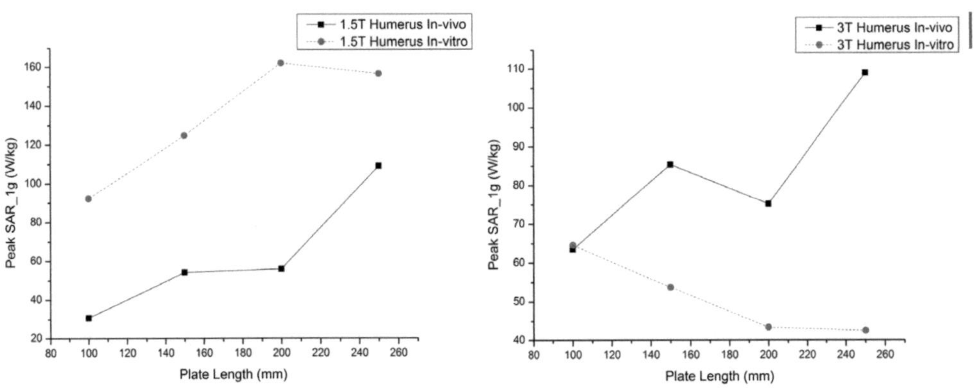

Figure 12. The humerus bone plate length study of 32 mm screw for 1.5 T (left) and 3 T (right).

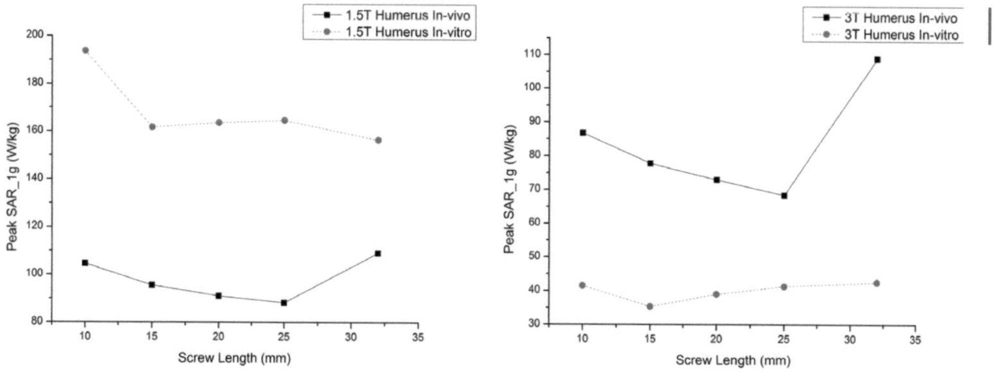

Figure 13. The humerus screw length study for 1.5 T (left) and 3 T (right).

4.3. Hip prostheses

For hip prostheses, the 1g average local peak SAR value at device is also extracted for each configuration. **Table 5** shows the value for hip system of various dimensions. The height of hip prostheses stem ranges from 100 to 170 mm. For *in-vivo* simulation, the stem is inserted into the bone marrow. And for the trochanter region, the hip prostheses is touching with soft tissue and muscle. **Figure 14** represents the results of hip prostheses. The solid and dash curve and indicate the *in-vivo* and *in-vitro* results, respectively.

4.4. Tibia intramedullary nails

The 1g average local peak SAR value at device is also extracted for each configuration of tibia intramedullary nails. The length of stem ranges from 255 to 360 mm. The entire nail

Stem height (mm)	1.5 T/64 MHz		3 T/128 MHz	
	In-vivo SAR_{1g} (W/kg)	*In-vitro* SAR_{1g} (W/kg)	*In-vivo* SAR_{1g} (W/kg)	*In-vitro* SAR_{1g} (W/kg)
100	83.2764	270.843	43.4746	55.4143
110	81.5782	260.502	35.8247	56.3111
120	77.8568	248.116	24.4627	57.0498
130	74.9259	247.635	21.9093	60.352
140	64.5142	237.51	16.3059	61.7026
150	62.8772	205.328	13.1482	63.2055
160	59.6273	221.781	11.5599	63.9114
170	55.0469	213.602	11.1877	63.8915

Table 5. Peak 1g average SAR of hip prostheses system for *in-vivo* and *in-vitro* cases.

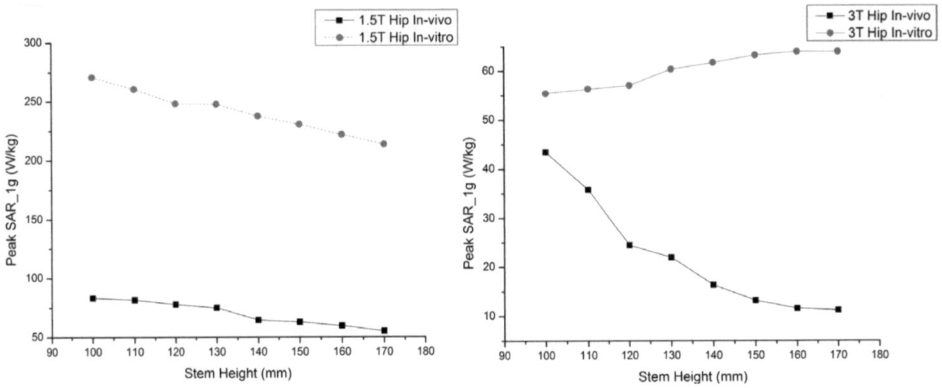

Figure 14. The hip prostheses stem length study for 1.5 T (left) and 3 T (right).

Nail length (mm)	1.5 T/64 MHz		3 T/128 MHz	
	In-vivo SAR_{1g} (W/kg)	*In-vitro* SAR_{1g} (W/kg)	*In-vivo* SAR_{1g} (W/kg)	*In-vitro* SAR_{1g} (W/kg)
255	77.6968	136.331	93.5532	55.4068
270	77.6346	129.249	93.2341	53.6038
285	78.9892	122.28	89.1767	49.8946
300	82.6751	115.745	91.5648	46.8385
315	81.7577	109.28	92.7346	44.0529
330	74.7444	103.319	88.9989	41.6544
345	66.6095	97.3232	90.7795	39.3275
360	67.3469	91.8168	90.1809	37.1875

Table 6. Peak 1g average SAR of tibia nails system for *in-vivo* and *in-vitro* cases.

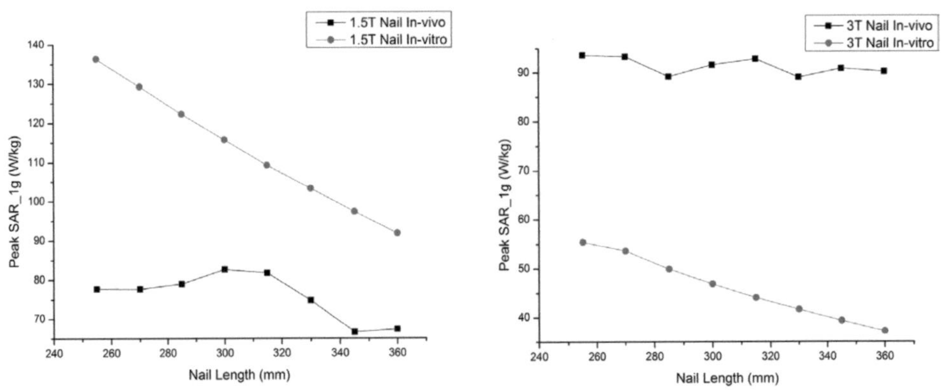

Figure 15. The nail length study for 1.5 T (left) and 3 T (right).

is penetrated into the bone marrow. The four screws are inserted perpendicularly through the nail and bone. **Table 6** shows the value for nail system of various dimensions. **Figure 15** represents the results of tibia intramedullary nails. The solid and dash curve and indicate the *in-vivo* and *in-vitro* results, respectively.

5. Summary

From the comparison between *in-vitro* and *in-vivo* simulations, the RF-induced heating are different because of the variance of incident electric field and surrounding medium. For incident field study, the antenna resonance effect would mainly lead to a heating issue for both *in-vitro* and *in-vivo* situation. Although the wavelength of human muscle and gelled-saline nearly equals to each other, due to the variance of incident RF field, the device dimension causing the resonance would be different. Hence, the trend of peak 1g average SAR value along with plate length is unlike from *in-vitro* to *in-vivo* circumstance. Additionally, when the screw is inserted across the human bone into the muscle, a huge amount of power would dissipated to the human tissue through the screw tip so that induce a large peak SAR value.

Based on the comparison result, conservatively, the *in-vitro* method, such as ASTM phantom, could be used to assess RF-induced heating. However, to accurately assess the RF-induced heating in heterogeneous human body with implantable medical device, due to the limit of homogeneous ASTM phantom, it still needs some improvement to handle several particular cases, especially, when the implantable device is penetrating through various human tissues and organs.

Disclaimer

The mention of commercial products, their sources, or their use in connection with material reported herein is not to be construed as either an actual or implied endorsement of such products by the Department of Health and Human Services.

Author details

Ran Guo, Jianfeng Zheng* and Ji Chen

*Address all correspondence to: jzheng4@central.uh.edu

Department of Electrical and Computer Engineering, University of Houston, Houston, Texas, United States

References

[1] Schenck JF. Health effects and safety of static magnetic fields. In: Shellock FG, editor. Magnetic Resonance Procedures: Health Effects and Safety. Boca Raton, FL: CRC; 2001. p. 1-30

[2] Zaremba LA. FDA guidance for magnetic resonance system safety and patient exposures: Current status and future considerations. In: Shellock FG, editor. Magnetic Resonance Procedures: Health Effects and Safety. Boca Raton, FL: CRC; 2001. p. 183-196

[3] U.S. Food and Drug Administration, Center for Devices and Radiological Health. MDR Data Files. Available at: www.fda.gov/CDRH/mdrfile.html. [Accessed: April 1, 2003]

[4] U.S. Food and Drug Administration, Center for Devices and Radiological Health. Manufacturer and User Facility Device Experience Database (MAUDE): File Formats for FOI Releasable Data. Available at: www.fda.gov/cdrh/maude.html

[5] Shellock FG. Reference Manual for Magnetic Resonance Safety, Implants, and Devices: 2004 Edition. Los Angeles, CA: Biomedical Research Publishing; 2004

[6] Shellock FG. Pocket Guide to MR Procedures and Metallic Objects: Update 2001. Philadelphia, PA: Lippincott Williams &Wilkins; 2001

[7] Shellock FG. Magnetic Resonance Procedure: Health Effects and Safety. Boca Raton, FL: CRC; 2001

[8] Edelman RR, Shellock FG, Ahladis J, Practical MRI. For the technologist and imaging specialist. In: Edelman RR, Hesselink J, editors. Clinical Magnetic Resonance. Philadelphia: WB Saunders; 1990. p. 80-115

[9] Persson BRR, Stahlberg F. Health and Safety of Clinical NMR Examinations. Boca Raton, FL: CRC Press; 1989. p. 59-79

[10] Shellock FG, Kanal E. Magnetic Resonance: Bio Effects, Safety, and Patient Management. 2nd ed. New York: Lippincott-Raven; 1996. p. 25-48

[11] Shellock FG. Biological effects and safety aspects of magnetic resonance imaging. Magnetic Resonance Quarterly. 1989;**5**:243-261

[12] Kanal E, Shellock FG, Talagala L. Safety considerations in MR imaging. Radiology. 1990; **176**:593-606

[13] Morvan D, Leroy-Willig A, Jehenson P, Cuenod CA, Syrota A. Temperature changes induced in human muscle by radiofrequency H-1 coupling: Measurement with an MR imaging diffusion technique. Radiology. 1992;**185**:871-874

[14] Shellock FG. MRI Bioeffects and safety. In: Atlas S, editor. Magnetic Resonance Imaging of the Brain and Spine. New York: Raven Press; 1990

[15] Shellock FG. Thermal responses in human subjects exposed to magnetic resonance imaging. Annals of the New York Academy of Sciences. 1992:260-272

[16] Bottomley PA, Redington RW, Edelstein WA, et al. Estimating radiofrequency power deposition in body NMR imaging. Magnetic Resonance in Medicine. 1985;**2**:336-349

[17] Bottomley PA, Edelstein WA. Power deposition in whole body NMR imaging. Medical Physics. 1981;**8**:510-512

[18] Shellock FG. Magnetic resonance imaging: bioeffects, safety, and patient management [J]. Reviews of Magnetic Resonance in Medicine. 1992;**4**:21-63

[19] Schaefer DJ, Barber BJ, Gordon CJ, et al. Thermal effects of magnetic resonance imaging. In: Book of Abstracts, Society for Magnetic Resonance in Medicine. Vol. 2. Berkeley, CA: Society for Magnetic Resonance in Medicine. 1985. p. 925

[20] Gordon CJ. Thermal physiology. In: Biological Effects of Radiofrequency Radiation. Washington, DC: EPA-600/8-83-026A; 1984 P 4-1-4-28

[21] Gordon CJ. Effect of radiofrequency radiation exposure on thermoregulation. ISI Atlas of Science, Animal and Plant Sciences. 1988;**1**:245-250

[22] Gordon CJ. Normalizing the thermal effects of radiofrequency radiation: Body mass versus total body surface area. Bioelectromagnetics. 1987;**8**:111-118

[23] ASTM International· Standard Test Method for Measurement of radio frequency induced heating near passive implants during magnetic resonance imaging ASTM Standard F2182-11. ASTM International: West Conshohocken, PA; 2011 www.astm.org

[24] Powell J, Papadaki A, Hand J, Hart A, McRobbie D. Numerical simulation of SAR induced around Co-Cr-Mo hip prostheses in situ expose to RF fields associated with 1.5 and 3 T MR body coils. Magnetic Resonance in Medicine. 2012;**68**:960-968

[25] Liu Y, Chen J, Shellock FG, et al. Computational and experimental studies of an orthopedic implant: MRI-related heating at 1.5-T/64-MHz and 3-T/128-MHz. Journal of Magnetic Resonance Imaging. 2013;**37**(2):491-497

[26] Liu Y, Shen J, Kainz W, et al. Numerical investigations of MRI RF field induced heating for external fixation devices. Biomedical Engineering Online. 2013;**12**(1):12

[27] Guo R, Zheng J, Chen J, et al. RF-induced heating comparison between *in-vivo* and in-phantom for 1.5 T MRI. Electromagnetic compatibility (EMC), 2016 IEEE International Symposium on IEEE, 2016: 121-125

[28] Mohsin SA, Sheikh NM, Abbas W. MRI induced heating of artificial bone implants. Journal of Electromagnetic Waves and Applications. 2009;**23**:799-808

[29] Li D, Zheng J, Liu Y, et al. An efficient approach to estimate MRI RF field induced in vivo heating for small medical implants. IEEE Transactions on Electromagnetic Compatibility. 2015;**57**(4):643-650

[30] Zheng J, Li D, Chen J, et al. Numerical study of SAR for multi-component orthopaedic hip replacement system during MRI. Electromagnetic Compatibility (EMC), 2016 IEEE International Symposium on IEEE, 2016: 116-120

[31] Zeng Q, Wang Q, Zheng J, et al. MRI induced heating for fully implanted, partially implanted and minimally implanted medical electrode leads. Electromagnetics in Advanced Applications (ICEAA), 2015 International Conference on IEEE, 2015: 1590-1591

[32] Zeng Q, Zheng J, Chen J. MRI Induced heating for fully implanted, partially implanted and minimum implanted medical electrode leads. Applied Computational Electromagnetics (ACES), 2015 31st International Review of Progress in IEEE, 2015:1-2

[33] Hand JW. Modelling the interaction of electromagnetic fields (10 MHz–10 GHz) with the human body: Methods and applications. Physics in Medicine and Biology. 2008;**53**(16):R243

[34] Andreo P. Monte Carlo techniques in medical radiation physics. Physics in Medicine and Biology. 1991;**36**(7):861

[35] Yee K. Numerical solution of initial boundary value problems involving Maxwell's equations in isotropic media. IEEE Transactions on Antennas and Propagation. 1966;**14**(3): 302-307

[36] Patankar SV. Numerical Heat Transfer and Fluid Flow. New York: Hemisphere; 1980. p. 25-73

[37] Christ A, Kainz W, Hahn EG, et al. The virtual family—Development of surface-based anatomical models of two adults and two children for dosimetric simulations. Physics in Medicine and Biology. 2009;**55**(2):N23

Chapter 6

Advanced Brain Tumour Segmentation from MRI Images

Kavitha Angamuthu Rajasekaran and
Chellamuthu Chinna Gounder

Additional information is available at the end of the chapter

http://dx.doi.org/10.5772/intechopen.71416

Abstract

Magnetic resonance imaging (MRI) is widely used medical technology for diagnosis of various tissue abnormalities, detection of tumors. The active development in the computerized medical image segmentation has played a vital role in scientific research. This helps the doctors to take necessary treatment in an easy manner with fast decision making. Brain tumor segmentation is a hot point in the research field of Information technology with biomedical engineering. The brain tumor segmentation is motivated by assessing tumor growth, treatment responses, computer-based surgery, treatment of radiation therapy, and developing tumor growth models. Therefore, computer-aided diagnostic system is meaningful in medical treatments to reducing the workload of doctors and giving the accurate results. This chapter explains the causes, awareness of brain tumor segmentation and its classification, MRI scanning process and its operation, brain tumor classifications, and different segmentation methodologies.

Keywords: magnetic resonance imaging, segmentation, classification, tumor, diagnostic system

1. Basics of medical research

Digital image processing is a multidisciplinary area used in medical sciences, microscopy, astronomy, computer vision, geology, and many other fields. Medical imaging is one of the most important aspects of scientific and medical research. It provides computerized medical-image segmentation and computer-aided design. Particularly, these enhancements in medical imaging lead to the improved planning and accuracy of surgical procedures using human-machine intervention. This brings the therapeutic plan and the development of imaging instruments to provide some of the most effective diagnostic tools in the medical field. Recently, many medical instruments have been developed to produce sectional views of the human anatomy. The two major non-invasive techniques used for imaging the human body are computed tomography (CT) and magnetic resonance imaging (MRI). The MRI is used as a medical diagnostic tool for studying the human anatomy and is based on the principles of nuclear magnetic resonance (NMR), to provide information about the properties of materials. The NMR was developed by Bloch and Purcell in the 1940s [1, 2]. In the year 1970, Paul Lautenberg, Ray Damadian, and Peter Mansfield began to use the principles of NMR in MRI as an imaging modality for the head, spine, and body. MRI produces images of high spatial resolution with good soft tissue contrast that has made it useful for the detection of diseases. In x, Paul Lauterbur and Peter Mansfield were awarded the Nobel Prize in Physiology or Medicine for their simultaneous pioneering research applying MRI to the human body [3].

1.1. Motivation for brain tumor segmentation

Brain tumor segmentation is one of the most important and difficult tasks in many medical-image applications because it usually involves a huge amount of data. Artifacts due to patient's motion, limited acquisition time, and soft tissue boundaries are usually not well defined. There are large class of tumor types which have variety of shapes and sizes. They may appear indifferent sizes and types with different image intensities. Some of them may also affect the surrounding structures that change the image intensities around the tumor.

Moreover, the World Health Organization (WHO) states that around 400,000 people in the world are affected with the brain tumor and 120,000 people have died in the previous year [4–7]. Before the treatment of chemotherapy, radiotherapy, or brain surgeries, there is a need for medical practitioners to confirm the boundaries and regions of the brain tumor and determine where exactly it is located and the exact affected area. For reviewing the adverse effects of the cancer, the tool can be automatic or semi-automatic for brain tumor segmentation can helps and also acts as a pre-requisite stage for doctors to identify the brain tumor before performing surgeries.

1.2. Magnetic resonance imaging (MRI)

The MRI is a diagnostic tool used for analyzing and studying the human anatomy. Huang [8], Zhan et al. [9], and Yang et al. [10] explained the medical images acquired in various bands of the electromagnetic spectrum. The wide variety of sensors used for the acquisition of images and the physics behind them, make each modality suitable for a specific purpose.

In MRI, the pictures are produced using a magnetic field, which is approximately 10,000 times stronger than the earth's magnetic field (Armstrong [11], Stark [6], and Steen [7]). The MRI produces more detailed images than other techniques, such as CT or ultrasound. The MRI also provides maps of anatomical structures with a high soft-tissue contrast. Basically, the magnetic resonance of hydrogen (1H) nuclei in water and lipid is measured by an MRI scanner. As the signal values are 12-bit coded, 4096 shades can be represented by a pixel [11]. The MRI scanners require a magnetic field and it is available at 1.5 or 3 T. In comparison with the earth's magnetic field (~50 μT) the magnetic field of a 3 T MRI scanner is approximately 60,000 times the earth field. The patient is placed in a strong magnetic field, which causes the protons in the water molecules of the body to align either in a parallel or anti-parallel orientation with the magnetic field. A radiofrequency pulse is introduced, causing the spinning protons to move out of the alignment. When the pulse is stopped, the protons realign and emit radio frequency energy signal that is localized by the magnetic fields and are spatially varied and rapidly turned on and off. A radio antenna within the scanner detects the signal and creates the image. Terms used in MRI are shown in **Table 1**.

MR-based imaging techniques are used to characterize the brain tumor according to their anatomy and physiology. Clinicians, particularly are interested in determining tumor location, extent, amount of necrosis, vascular supply, and associated edema. There are different imaging techniques that are useful in providing a relevant differential diagnosis. The various techniques used today for imaging brain tumor are contrast agents, fat suppression, MR angiography, functional MRI, diffusion weighted imaging (DWI), MR spectroscopy, and fast fluid-attenuated inversion-recovery (FLAIR). Different methods of imaging are applied in the clinical environment according to tumor type and diagnostic requirements. The methods used in the diagnosis work are described in detail [8, 12].

The contrast agents technique delivers an excellent soft-tissue contrast. Sometimes there is a need to administer exogenous contrast usually an intravenous injection of some paramagnetic agent, most commonly Gd-DTPA. The effect of this agent is to shorten the relaxation time of local spins causing a decrease in signal on T2-weighted images and an increase on T1-weighted images. The MRI brain image before and after contrast enhancement is shown in **Figure 1**.

The increased vascularity of tumors produces a preferential uptake of contrast agent and it can be used to better observe the tumors from the surrounding normal tissue. If MRI scans are repeatedly acquired following the contrast injection, the dynamic nature of contrast uptake can be examined, which may improve the differentiation of benign and malignant disease.

MR angiography is one of the biggest growth areas of MRI. In normal circumstances, the flow effects can cause unwanted artifacts. But, in MRA these phenomena are used advantageously to permit the non-invasive imaging of the vascular tree. Techniques can be generally divided into "white" or "black" blood methods depending on whether moving spins appear brighter

Term	Description
T1	The time needed for the protons in the tissue to return to their original state of magnetization
T2	The time required for the protons perturbed into coherent oscillation by the radiofrequency pulse to loosen this coherence
TR	Repetition time: the time between successive applications of radiofrequency pulse sequences
TE	Echo time: the delay before the radiofrequency energy radiated by the tissue in question is measured
T1-weighted image	Short TR, short TE. Provides better anatomic detail
T2-weighted image	Long TR, short TE. More sensitive to water content and as a result, more sensitive to pathology
FLAIR image	Long TR, short TE. Improved contrast between lesions and cerebrospinal fluid

Table 1. Summaries of terms used in MRI.

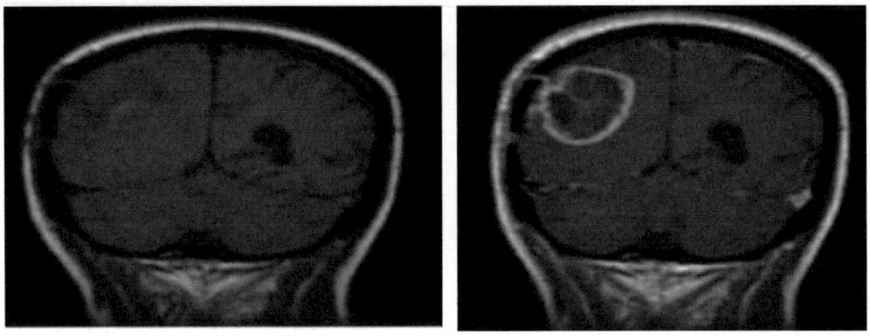

Figure 1. MRI image contrast enhancement. (a) Before (b) after.

or darker than the stationary tissue. In high-velocity signal loss, the blood that has moved in-between 90 and 180° pulses will not produce a signal and will appear dark. If a short TR is used, the spins in the imaging slice become quickly saturated and "fresh" spins flowing into this slice have their full magnetization available to emit a high signal. This technique works the best way over thin sections when blood flow is perpendicular to the imaging plane. Although current clinical agents are extracellular, they quickly distribute into the extra vascular space and the accurate timing of imaging sequence following the contrast injection can provide excellent results. Good timing of arterial bolus with the center of k-space acquisition is crucial to avoid artifacts. This can be achieved by using a small "test bolus" or by monitoring the contrast flow using rapid 2D images before initiating the real imaging sequence. The angiography provided by MRI imaging is shown in **Figure 2**.

Functional MRI is a technique for examining the brain activation, which unlike PET, is non-invasive with relatively high spatial resolution. The most common method utilizes a technique called blood oxygen level dependent contrast. This is an example of endogenous contrast, making use of the inherent signal differences in blood oxygenation content. In the normal resting state, a high concentration of deoxyhemoglobin attenuates the MRI signal due to its paramagnetic nature. However, the neuronal activity, in response to some task or stimulus, creates a local demand for the oxygen supply, which increases the fraction of oxy hemoglobin causing a signal increase on T2 or T2*-weighted images. In a typical experiment, the patient is subjected to a series of rest and task intervals, during which MRI images are repeatedly acquired. The signal changes during the course of time are then examined on a pixel-by-pixel basis to test how well they correlate with the known stimulus pattern. The pixels that demonstrate a statistically significant correlation are highlighted in color and overlaid onto a gray-scale MRI image to create an activation map of the brain. The location and extent of activation is linked to the type of stimulus. Thus, a simple thumb-finger movement task will produce activation in the primary motor cortex. The functional study and activation map of MRI is shown in **Figure 3**.

Diffusion-weighted imaging is an MRI technique, in which contrast within the image is based on the movement of the water molecules. The diffusion refers to the random motion of the molecules along a concentration gradient. The diffusion-weighted MRI is another example of

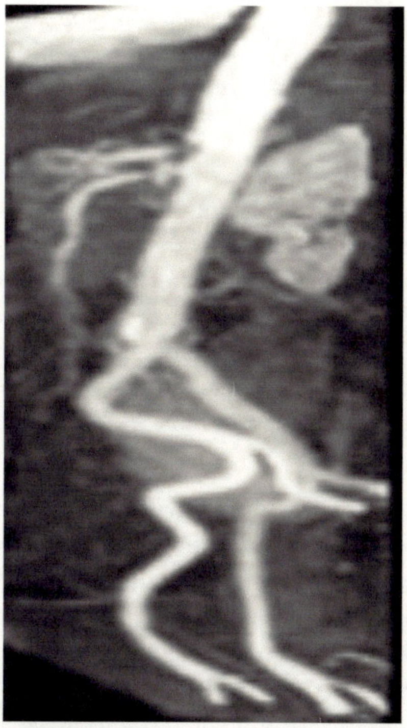

Figure 2. MRI angiography (Courtesy: Siemens.com).

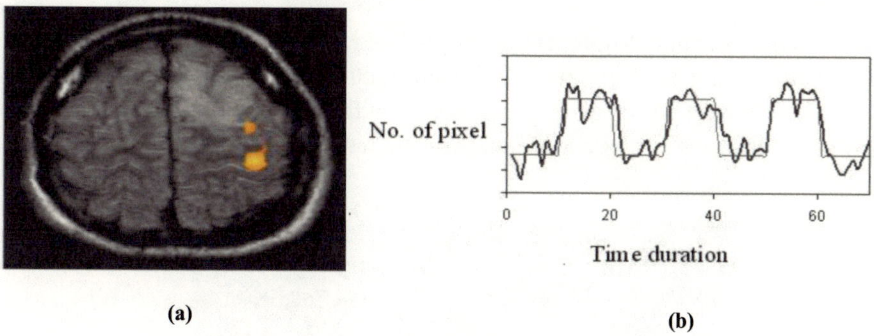

Figure 3. Functional study of MRI. (a) MRI image (b) activation map of the MRI image.

endogenous contrast, using the motion of spins to produce signal changes. The most common method employs the Stejskal-Tanner bipolar gradient scheme. The gradients with equal amplitude, but opposite polarity, are applied over a given interval. The stationary tissue is dephased and rephased equally, whereas the spins which have moved during the interval suffer a net dephasing and signal loss. By using gradients of sufficiently high amplitude, the sequence is made sensitive to the motion at the microscopic level. The signal attenuation depends on the degree of diffusion, the strength, and the timing of the gradients. By acquiring the images with different values of b factor, a value for the apparent diffusion coefficient can be calculated. The experiment is performed using diffusion gradients in any direction. However, to obtain a complete three-dimensional description of the diffusion, a tensor is calculated based on a new gradient image and combinations of gradient pairs. This is able to discern anisotropy due to preferential diffusion along the structures or fibers. The white matter tracts in a normal MRI brain image are shown in **Figure 4**.

MRI spectroscopy is a technique for displaying the metabolic information from an image. It relies on the inherent differences in the resonant frequency. The MRI signal is measured and a spectrum is displayed. By using a standard reference, the chemical species of each peak are determined. For proton MRI signal, the reference compound is tetramethylsilane. All the chemical shifts are expressed as the frequency differences from this compound giving a field-independent part per million scales. In this standard, the water has characteristic peak value of 4.7 ppm. Most methods use the intersection of three slice-select RF pulses to excite a volume of interest called a voxel.

The multiple voxels can be acquired by using phase encoding in each of the desired dimensions. This technique, called chemical shift imaging, is useful in isolating individual peaks and displaying the integrated area as a color scale to produce a metabolic map. The spectrum when acquired from a normal healthy brain tissue displays the characteristic peak signal defined as NAA; it provides images with excellent soft-tissue contrast. If a spectrum is taken from a slightly enlarged, but otherwise normal looking, part of the medulla, it does not show any enhancement with gadolinium. In this case, the NAA (*N-acetyl-aspartate*) peak is absent indicating the loss of viable tissue, and the choline peak is elevated indicating the high cell proliferation in tumors. The single voxel proton MRI of brain in normal and malignant tissue is shown in **Figure 5**.

The MRI images are dependent upon the absorption of radio waves by the hydrogen nuclei, 1H which has an intrinsic nuclear spin in sufficient quantities to enable the production of a useful image of the human body. Many of the protons within the human body are found in the nuclei of water. The generation of MRI images is a result of the sophisticated interaction

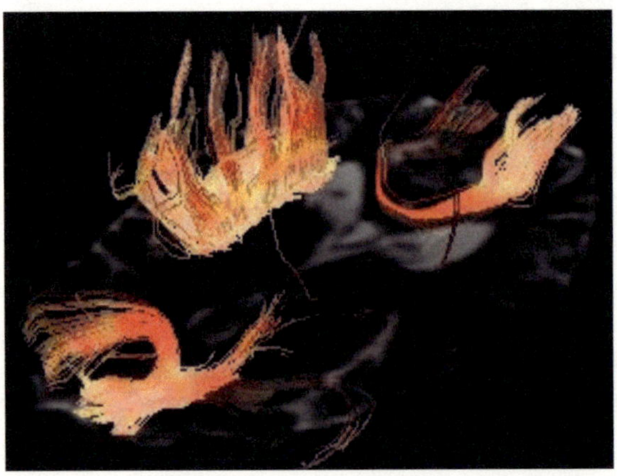

Figure 4. White matter tracks in a normal MRI brain image.

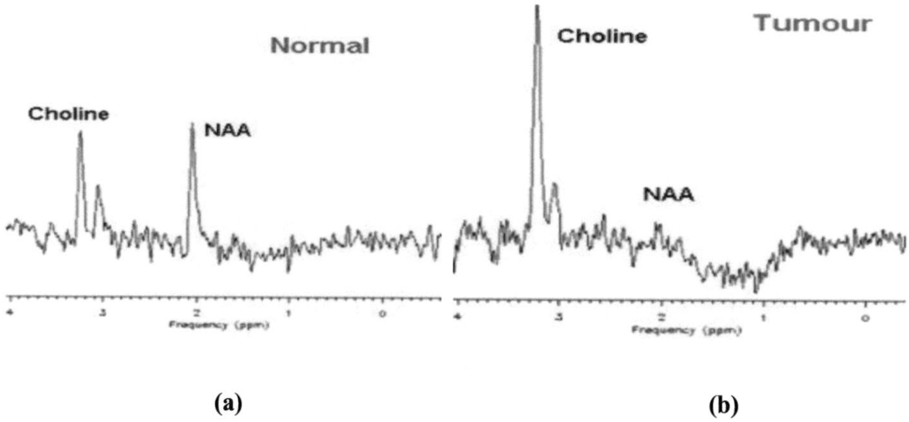

Figure 5. Single voxel proton MRI brain in normal and malignant tissue. (a) Normal (b) With tumour.

between the electronic components, radiofrequency generators, coils, and gradient that interface with a computer for communication between the different electronics. The magnet, gradient coils, and RF coils present in the MRI scanner are the basic parts that help to form an image. The schematic diagram of MRI scanner and the basic parts of the MRI scanner are shown in **Figure 6** [9, 13].

The magnet is used to form the "external" magnetic field in which the patient or object is placed. Three types of magnets can be used in MR imaging: permanent, resistive, and superconducting. The superconducting magnets are the most commonly used in the recent MRI scanners. The superconducting magnets with field strength 1.5–3.0 T range offer good image contrast due to the energy exchange between the protons and their environments.

The hydrogen proton is the primary nucleus used for MRI because it produces the strongest signal. Proton in the absence of an external magnetic field may be oriented along any direction. In the absence of an external magnetic field, the net magnetization vector will be zero. When placed in a strong external magnetic field the magnetic moments of the proton orient themselves along the magnetic flux lines. The magnetic moments of the protons align along the direction of actual magnetic field B_0. The equilibrium value of the magnitude of proton magnetization M_0 in the presence of magnetic field is given in Eq (1).

$$M_0 = \frac{N\gamma^2 h^2 I(I+1)B_0}{3kT_s} \tag{1}$$

where B_0 is the static magnetic field, N is the number of proton spins per unit volume, γ is the gyro magnetic ratio, a constant unique for each nucleus, h is the Planck's constant, I is the proton spin, T_s is the absolute sample temperature in Kelvin, and k is the Boltzmann's constant.

Thus, the magnetization M_0 is proportional to the external magnetic field B_0. The magnetic moments exhibit the property of processing around the field B_0. The Larmor frequency in MRI refers to the rate of precession of spin under the influence of magnetic moment of the proton around the external magnetic field. The precession of Larmor frequency f_L is given in Eq (2).

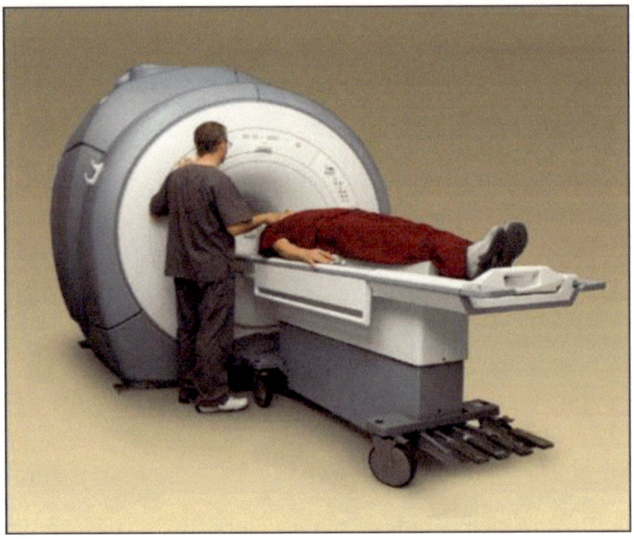

(a)

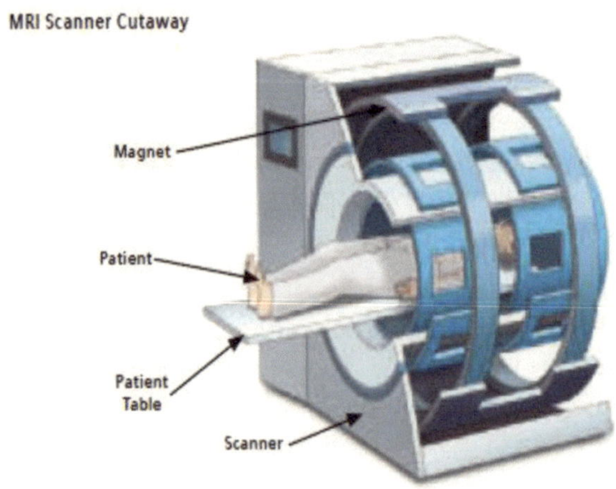

(b)

Figure 6. View of MRI scanner and the basic parts of MRI scanner. (a) The schematic diagram of MRI scanner (b) basic parts of the MRI scanner.

$$f_L = \frac{\gamma B_0}{2\pi} \tag{2}$$

For the proton, $\frac{\gamma}{2\pi}$ is equal to 42.58 MHz/Tesla. The Larmor frequency will be in the radio frequency region (40–50 MHz).

To obtain an MRI signal, the radio frequency (RF) pulses are applied at the Larmor frequency f_L perpendicular to the main magnetic field B_0 disturbing the magnetic moments of the protons

http://dx.doi.org/10.5772/intechopen.71416

from their equilibrium position. The protons are aligned along the static magnetic field. This alignment is disturbed by a 90° RF pulse and the total displacement is proportional to the RF-pulse energy and also the Larmor frequency. If the energy of the RF pulse is sufficient to tip the magnetization vector (M) by 90°, then it is tipped into the transverse plane. The magnetization vector continues to spinning process about B_0 in the transverse plane. The time-varying magnetization induces flux changes, which are detected in the RF coil. The relaxation constants are the important parameters of MRI. The MRI slice data are generated using an X-ray source that rotates around the object. The earliest sensors were scintillation detectors, with photo multiplier tubes excited by cesium iodide crystals. Cesium iodide was replaced during the 1980s by ion chambers containing high pressure xenon gas [14]. These systems were, in turn, replaced by scintillation systems based on the photo diodes, instead of photo multipliers. Many data scans are progressively taken, as the object is gradually passed through the gantry. The typical MRI system with the schematic diagram of MRI equipment mainly consists of five parts: the main magnet, gradient systems, RF system, computer systems, and other auxiliary equipment as shown in **Figure 7**.

The direction selection for MRI slices and MRI scan protocol [15, 16] for brain tumor patients are shown in **Figure 8** and **Table 2**.

In the MRI scanner, a section of the slice perpendicular to the z-axis is called axial plane. The plane that divides the brain into left and right parts is known as sagittal or median plane. The vertical plane that divides the brain into posterior and anterior parts is known as coronal or frontal plane. The MRI brain image in different planes is shown in the **Figure 9**.

MRI pixel representation mainly in order to increase the contrast between pathology and healthy tissue, enhancement agents such as gadolinium (Gd) may be used (Kim et al. 2013). The Gd has a large magnetic moment, which triggers fluctuations in the local magnetic field near the Larmor frequency. The MRI images are grids of pixels with 512 rows and 512

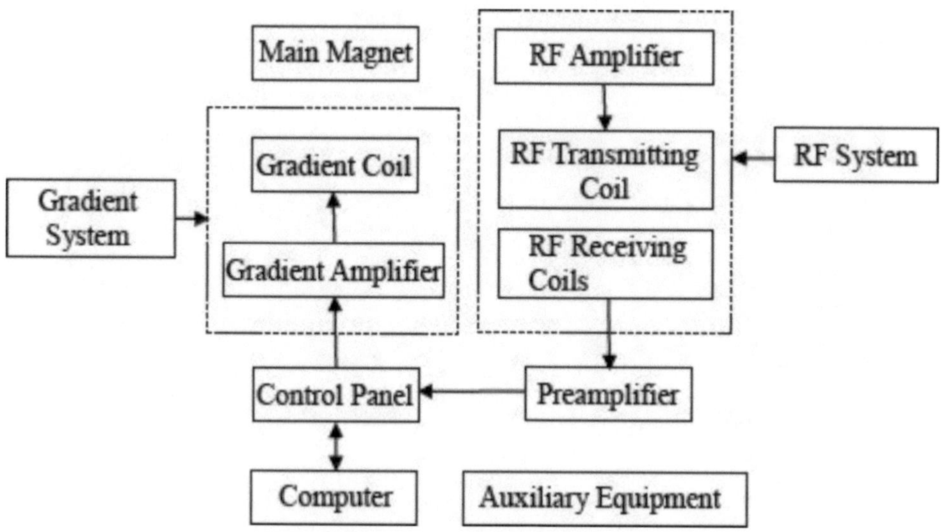

Figure 7. The schematic diagram of MRI equipment and MRI scan process.

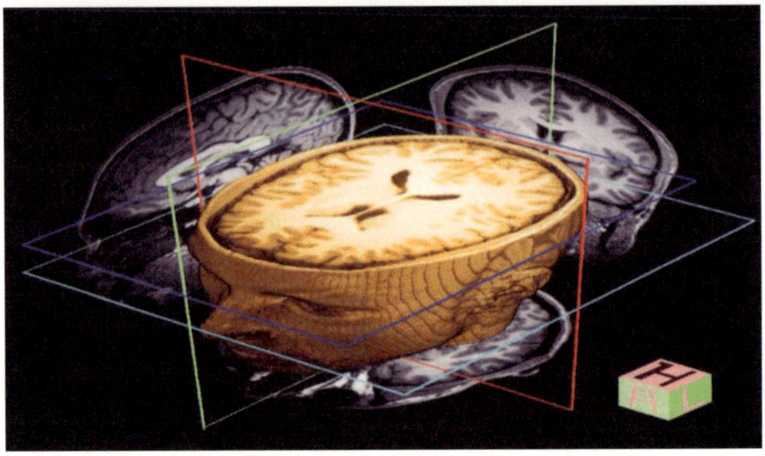

Sagittal, axial, coronal

Figure 8. The direction selection in MRI slices.

Anatomical plane	Weighting	Contrast	Slice thickness/spacing between slices (in mm)
Sagittal	T1-Weighted	–	5/6
Axial	T1-Weighted	–	4/4
Axial	T2-weighted	–	5/6
Axial	T2-weightedFLAIR	–	5/6
Axial	T1-Weighted	Gadolinium	4/4
coronal	T1-Weighted	Gadolinium	4/4
Sagittal	T1-Weighted	Gadolinium	5/6

Table 2. MRI scan protocol for brain tumor patients [15].

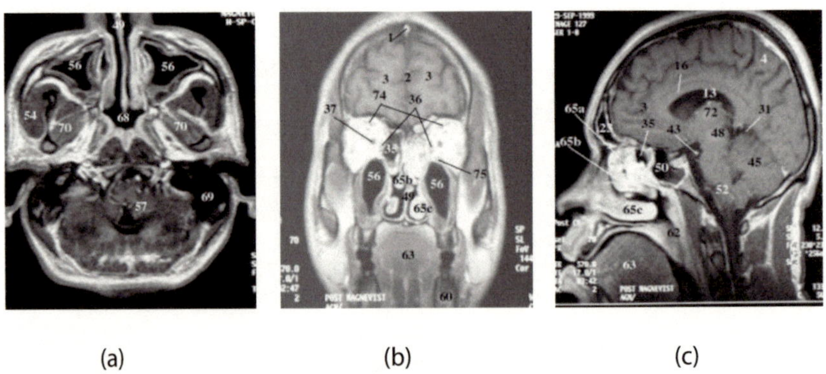

Figure 9. MRI brain image in different planes. (a) Axial (b) Coronal (c) Sagittal.

columns. Every pixel of an MRI image corresponds to a voxel, a volume element, whose value represents the tissue and MRI signal. The volume of a voxel depends on the MRI scan parameters like slice thickness and pixel spacing. The MRI images are usually delivered in DICOM format. Besides the brain image, the DICOM-files contain information about the scan and the patient. Normally, an MRI scan acquires more than one slice, which leads to an image sequence with 5.5 mm spacing between the slices [17]. The sequence of MRI for 256 slices is shown in **Figure 10** with 5.5 mm spacing between the slices.

In this thesis, the segmentation algorithm is applied to the MRI brain images with tumors. In order to understand the clinically important characteristics of the tumor tissues, the anatomy of brain is considered in the next section.

1.3. Anatomy of the brain classification of brain tumor

World Health Organization (WHO) classifies the brain tumors as: astrocytoma, low grade astrocytoma (grades I and II), high grade astrocytoma (grades III and IV), ganglioglioma, oligodendroglioma, ependymoma, and medulloblastoma.

The higher the grade, the more malignant is the tumor. The tumor grading helps the doctor, patient, and caregivers/family members to understand the patient's condition [18]. It also helps the doctor to plan treatment and predict outcome.

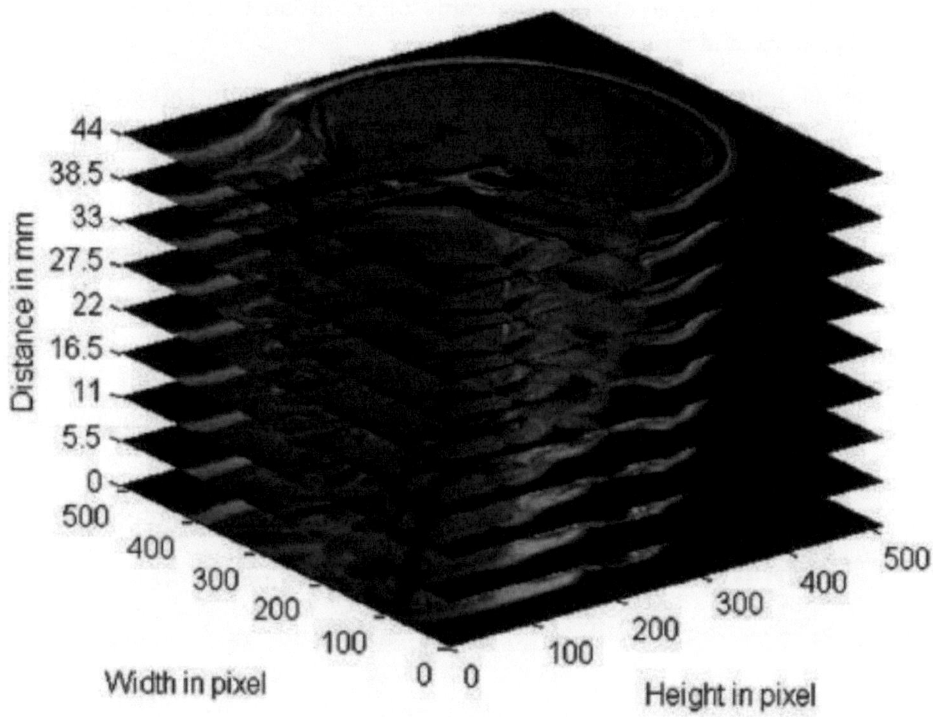

Figure 10. MRI sequence with 5.5 mm spacing between slices.

Grade-I is indicative of the least malignant tumors and is usually associated with long-term survival. These tumors grow slowly and have an almost normal appearance when viewed through a microscope. Only surgery may be required as an effective treatment for this grade tumor [19]. Pilocytic astrocytoma, craniopharyngioma, and other tumors of neurons such as gangliocytoma and ganglioglioma are the examples of grade I tumors.

Grade II tumors are slow-growing and look slightly abnormal under a microscope. Some can spread into nearby normal tissue and recur sometimes as a higher grade tumor.

Grade III tumors are, by definition, malignant although there is not always a big difference between grade II and grade III tumors. The cells of a grade III tumor are actively reproducing abnormal cells, which grow into nearby normal brain tissue. These tumors tend to recur often as a grade IV.

Grade IV are the most malignant tumors. They can have a bizarre appearance when viewed under the microscope, and easily grow into nearby normal brain tissue. These tumors form new blood vessels so that they can maintain their rapid growth. They also have areas of dead cells in their centers. The glioblastoma multiform is the most common example of a grade IV tumor. A sample of astrocytoma is (cite [20]) shown in **Figure 11**.

There are three classifications of tumors based on their location: local tumors, regional tumors, and distant tumors. The local tumors are confined to one hemisphere in one part of the brain, meninges, and ventricular system. The regional tumor crosses the midline or tentorium and invades bone, blood vessel, nerves, and spinal cord [16]. The distant tumors extend to the nasal cavity, nasal pharynx, and posterior pharynx.

Classification of tumors based on their radiological appearance includes non-enhanced tumors, full-enhanced tumors without edema, full-enhanced tumors with edema, and ring-enhanced tumors. Classification of tumors based on their alter-At ions consists of small deforming tumors (SD) and large deforming tumors (LD).

Brain tumor is diagnosed when a brain tumor is suspected; a doctor can carry out a number of tests to reach a diagnosis. These tests will help the doctor to determine the kind of tumor in the brain.

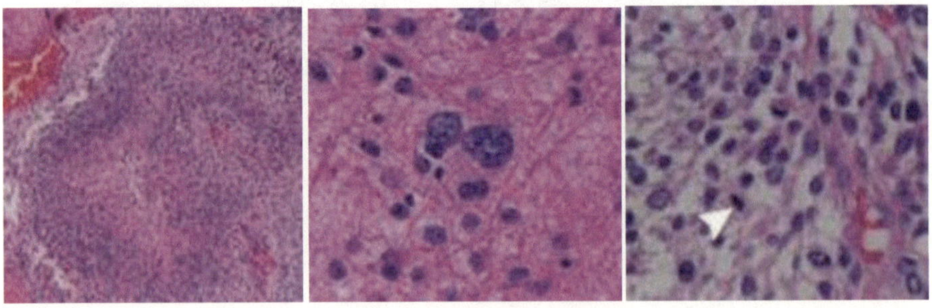

(a) **(b)** **(c)**

Figure 11. Sample of astrocytoma. (a)Astrocytoma IV (b) Astrocytoma II (c)Astrocytoma III.

http://dx.doi.org/10.5772/intechopen.71416

Some of the tests are performed first to diagnose the tumor and the results are used later to monitor the progress to determine whether the tumor has disappeared, is shrinking, remaining the same, or has changed in some way. Like many other medical conditions, the follow-up care for a brain tumor might go on for years.

The brain tumor diagnosis [16] is executed based on the Neurological Exam, Types of brain scans, X-rays, Laboratory test, DNA profiling, Biopsy procedure, and Tumor grading and staging.

A neurological exam includes a series of tests and procedures used to assess a person's nerves, senses, muscle strength, reflexes, balance, and mental state. The purpose of a neurological exam is to help the doctor determine the cause of the symptoms that brought the patient into the clinic in the first place.

MRI scans generate images of the brain for the purpose of diagnosing the tumor. The most common scans for diagnosis and follow-up are: MRI, CT, FMRI, dynamic MRI, angiography and MRI angiography MRS, positron emission tomography, single photon emission computerized tomography, and magneto encephalography.

The genetic profiling, or DNA profiling, is a lab test used to determine the specific features of patient DNA. It is a relatively new procedure that can give the doctor detailed information about the tumor. This information is used to develop a more specialized course of treatment, which may significantly increase the odds of success. A biopsy is a surgical procedure, in which a small amount of tumor tissue is removed and sent to a lab for evaluation. The purpose of a biopsy is to establish whether an image is cancerous or not. The biopsy can be performed as part of the surgery to remove a tumor, or as a separate procedure. In either case, the surgeon removes a small amount of tumor tissue and sends it to a lab for a pathologist to review. Three types of biopsy are often performed in patients with brain tumors. These include needle biopsy, stereotactic biopsy, and open biopsy. If the results of patient's biopsy are not normal, the patient goes back to the doctor for further tests and advice.

1.4. Brain tumor segmentation

A lot of research has been carried out in the area of segmentation. Various segmentation techniques are addressed in this survey. The content of this survey comprises three important contributions: fuzzy C-means (FCM), region growing (RG), and genetic-based methods. The aim is to study and identify of the suitable segmentation for MRI images. This above said aim is to grasp the characteristics of tumors in the patients, automatically segment the tumor, and assist the doctors in assessing the effects of treatment with clinical pathology analysis and improving the therapeutic treatment in the next pathological periods.

1.4.1. Image segmentation using fuzzy C-means (FCM) method

The fuzzy C-means method description and some of the recent researches for segmentation based on genetic methodologies are as follows:

The FCM is the most widespread clustering algorithm [21, 22], but it is more sensitive to initial cluster centers and easy to fall into the local minimum value, so that the global optimal solution cannot be obtain due to the local search hill-climbing method. The traditional FCM for image segmentation directly performs the clustering for pixel sample sets with an obvious disadvantage of computational complexity. So, it is very important to choose better initial cluster centers. If we choose better initial cluster centers, algorithm can converge to the real cluster centers quickly. The FCM algorithm is successfully applied in many real world problems such as astronomy, geology, medical imaging, target recognition, and image segmentation. FCM segmentation method has considerable benefits, because it could retain much more information from the original image than hard segmentation method [23]. The FCM algorithm is composed of the following steps:

1. Initialize

$$\mathrm{U} = \left[u_{ij}\right] \text{ matrix, } U^{(0)} \tag{3}$$

2. At k-step: calculate the centers vectors $c^{(k)} = \left[c_j\right]$ with $U^{(k)}$

$$c_{ij} = \frac{\sum_{i=1}^{N} u_{ij}^m x_j}{\sum_{i=1}^{N} u_{ij}^m} \tag{4}$$

3. Update $U^{(k)}, U^{(k+1)}$

$$U_{ij} = \frac{1}{\sum_{i=1}^{c}\left(\frac{\|x_i - c_j\|}{\|x_i - c_k\|}\right)^{\frac{2}{m-1}}} \tag{5}$$

4. If $\|U^{(k+1)} - U^{(k)}\| < \in$ then STOP; otherwise return to step 2.

u_{ij} is between 0 and 1, c_i denotes the centroids of cluster I, d_{ij} is the Euclidean distance between i^{th} centroid and j^{th} data point, m Є [1, ∞] is a weighting function.

This iteration will stop when $\max_{ij}\left\{|u_{ij}^{(k+1)} - u_{ij}^{(k)}|\right\} < \in$ where $\in$ is a termination criterion between 0 and 1, whereas k denotes the iteration steps. This procedure converges to a local minimum or a saddle point of j_m.

FCM algorithm is a minimization operation method of iterative optimization, which needs to repeat the calculation of membership and update value of U_{ij} and V_i. If image data n is quite huge, it meets the problem of heavy calculation burden and problem to assign the initial clusters. Therefore IFCM is proposed [24] as a new center initialization algorithm for measuring the initial centers. The implementation of IFCM is presented in this chapter.

Caldairou et al. [25] described the membership function for calculating the centroids of clusters. The membership function indicates the degree of the elements belonging to a specific class. The same element can belong to various categories in different levels and the sum of the corresponding values of all the membership functions is 1. The element that is determined belongs to a category which has the largest value of the membership function. This is the classification criterion used in the FCM-based algorithms. But, the algorithm is still sensitive to the initial cluster centers.

Hema Rajini et al. [24] proposed an enhanced k-means and improved kernelised FCM with improved cluster center initialization algorithm to segment the MRI brain images. The method selected the initial center used by the center initialization algorithm. This algorithm was based on maximum measure of the distance function which was found for cluster center detection process. The validity of clustering results was obtained using silhouette method and the results were compared with those of original k-means and FCM algorithms. The addition of post-processing technique to extract the tumor in MRI brain image could improve the detection of brain tumor results.

Zou Kaiqil et al. [22] proposed an IFCM algorithm for color image segmentation. It was proposed to solve the problem of heavy calculating burden and the disadvantage of clustering performance affected by initial cluster centers for FCM. The quick subtractive clustering (QSC) was used for getting initial cluster centers of the image data points. In order to reduce the computational complexity, the mapping from pixel space to Eigen vector space was used for modifying the object function. The algorithm was limited to only for the general image segmentation process and further a post-processing improvement was needed for detecting tumor in MRI images.

Yongmin Kim et al. [26] discussed a novel segmentation procedure. In this method, the segmentation played a crucial role in numerous biomedical imaging applications, assisting clinicians or medical professionals to diagnose various diseases using scientific data. It required high computational time which limited its applicability.

William Sandham et al. [27] proposed a FCM segmentation of MRI brain image using neighborhood attraction with neural-network optimization. In this method, the updating process combined the classified elements and the membership functions instead of the traditional operations which rely on the data points. If the MRI image contains noise or is affected by the presence of artifacts, it can change the pixel intensities leading to improper segmentation. These problems must be properly addressed to improve the updating of membership value of the FCM algorithm.

Maoguo Gong et al. [28] explained an FCM Clustering with local information and kernel metric for image segmentation. An IFCM algorithm for image segmentation introduced a tradeoff between weighted fuzzy factor and a kernel metric. The new algorithm adaptively determined the kernel parameter by using a fast bandwidth selection rule based on the distance variance of all the data points in the collection. The weighted fuzzy factor depended both on the distance of all the neighboring pixels and their gray-level difference. By using this factor, the new algorithm could accurately estimate the damping extent of the neighboring pixels.

Ref. [29] addressed the FCM algorithm for GBM brain tumor segmentation. They used T1-weighed, T2-weighted, and Proton Density(PD)-weighted MRI with a vectorial FCM to segment the pathological brain into white matter, gray matter, cerebral fluid, tumor, and edema. Although the FCM algorithm was simple, fast and unsupervised, it could not segment the tumor and edema accurately because of the intensities of the overlapping tissues. The FCM was very sensitive to noise and initialization values and it was validated and tested for limited cases.

Zulaikha Beevi et al. [30] presented a robust and efficient approach for the segmentation of noisy medical images. The proposed approach utilized the histogram-based FCM clustering algorithm for the segmentation of MRI brain images and the cluster density was focused. The heavy calculating burden was the drawback of this method.

In all the methods applied to the brain tumor segmentation, the partitioning of the data was carried out through a membership function at each iterative process. In the iterative process, the samples of the same groups were more similar to one another than the samples belonging to different groups. The major drawback of the FCM is that it is sensitive to the initialization problem due to noise, initial centers of clusters, and different sizes of tumor. The computational time is high for executing the segmentation process.

In all the above studies fuzzy C-means method and it steps for segmenting and detecting tumor of the MRI brain images are discussed.

1.4.2. Image segmentation using region growing (RG) method

The region growing methodology and recent related work of region growing are described here.

RG is a simple image segmentation method based on the seeds of region [31]. It is also classified as a pixel-based image segmentation method since it involves the selection of initial seed points. This approach to segmentation examines the neighboring pixels of initial "seed points" and determines whether the pixel neighbors should be added to the region or not based on certain conditions. In a normal region growing technique, the neighbor pixels are examined by using only the "intensity" constraint. A threshold level for intensity value is set and those neighbor pixels that satisfy this threshold is selected for the region growing. The processing steps are

- Select the initial seed point
- Append the neighboring pixels—intensity threshold
- Check threshold of the neighboring pixel
- Thresholds satisfy-selected for growing the region.
- Process is iterated to end of all regions.

Ref. [32] explained an automatic approach for segmenting the MRI images. The segmentation problem was formulated as a problem in region growing. In particular, the method started locally by searching for a seed region of the left atrium from an MRI slice. A global constraint was imposed by applying a shape prior to the representation of left atrium by Zernike moments. The planning and evaluation procedures of left atriumablation were commonly based on the segmentation of the left atrium which was a challenging task due to large anatomical variations.

Yunliang Cai et al. [33] carried out detecting, grouping, and structure inference for invariant repetitive patterns in the images. Repetitive patterns are products of repetitive structures, repetitive reflections, or color patterns. The segmentation algorithm proposed in this paper followed the classical region growing image segmentation scheme. It utilized a mean-shift-like dynamic process to group the local image patches into clusters. It exploited a continuous joint alignment to match similar patches and refined the subspace grouping. The result of higher level grouping of image patterns could be used to infer the geometry of objects and estimate the general layout of a crowded scene.

Shafaf Ibrahim et al. [31] presented a comparison of segmentation algorithm performances between three techniques of seed-based region growing (SBRG), adaptive network-based fuzzy inference system (ANFIS), and FCM paradigms. All the three methods were found to be promising for segmentation of light abnormalities. Nevertheless, the segmentation performances of dark abnormalities were observed to produce moderate significances of correlation values in all conditions. These resulted in the segmentation of dark abnormalities becoming not as good as the segmentation in light abnormalities.

Nigri Happ et al. [34] presented a region growing segmentation algorithm for parallel version of graphics processing units. This method widely used by the geographic object-based image analysis. Initially, all the image pixels were considered as seeds or primitive segments. The fine-grained parallel threads assigned to the individual pixels merged the adjacent pixels iteratively and ensured that the increase in heterogeneity was minimized. The accuracy of the segmentation is low based on this approach.

Aman Chandra Kaushik et al. [35] proposed a content-based active contour method (CBAC) using both intensity and texture information present within the active contour. It also used a Gray-Level Co-occurrence Matrix (GLCM) to define texture space for tumor segmentation in MATLAB. The region growing method was used for segmenting ROI and edge detection by utilizing the boundary segmentation. The main drawback of this method was under segmentation and over segmentation.

Bhoi and Meher [36] presented a method for the removal of Gaussian noise for MRI images. It performed well in terms of peak signal to noise ratio (PSNR) over many well-known spatial and wavelet domain methods. The method also retained the edges beside the region growing methods for segmenting the MRI brain images.

Bhandarkar and Nammalwar [37] investigated the application of a hierarchical self-organizing map (HSOM) to the problem of segmentation of multispectral MRI images. The HSOM was composed of several layers of self-organizing maps (SOMs) organized in a pyramidal fashion. SOMs were used for the segmentation of multispectral MRI images, but the results often suffer from under segmentation or over segmentation.

James Tilton [38] described an approach for producing high quality hierarchically related image segmentation method. The hierarchically related image segmentations were at different levels in which the less-detailed segmentations could be produced from specific region merging algorithm. The region merging based hierarchical segmentation (HSEG) was presented, along with its recursive hierarchical segmentation (RHSEG). It was applied for exploiting the information content from the segmentation hierarchy based on changes in the region features. The seed point selection in the hierarchical segmentation as well as recursive hierarchical segmentation was still challenging in this approach.

Jabbar et al. [39] explained the major role of the image segmentation in biomedical imaging applications such as the enumeration of tissue volume diagnosis, confinement of pathology analysis of anatomical structure, treatment planning, partial volume improvement of practical imaging data, and computer incorporated surgery.

Jaya et al. [40] explained that the tumor types and classification of the tumor could straightforwardly wipe out all the fit brain cells. They explained the detail survey about the brain tumor and explained the effect of brain tumor. They also explained the brain tumor strong cells by crowding further parts of the brain and bringing about inflammation, brain swelling, and pressure inside the skull.

Jue Wu et al. [41] proposed a framework for multi-object segmentation of deep brain structures, which have significant shape variations and relatively small sizes in medical brain images. The method suggested a template-based framework, which fused the information of edge features, region statistics, and inter-structure constraints to detect and locate all the targeted brain structures. The multi-object template was organized in the form of a hierarchical Markov dependence tree. It was applicable for multi-object segmentation of deep brain structures (caudate nucleus, putamen, and thalamus) in the MRI brain images.

Kekre et al. [42] presented a vector quantization segmentation method to detect cancerous mass from MRI images. In order to increase the radiologist's diagnostic performance, a computer-aided diagnosis scheme was developed to improve the detection of primary signatures of these diseased masses and micro-classifications.

Corso et al. [43] presented a method for automatic segmentation of heterogeneous image data where the Bayesian formulation was included to incorporate the soft model assignments for calculating affinities.

Liao et al. [44] proposed a fast spatially constrained kernel clustering algorithm for segmentation which corrected the intensity in homogeneities for the MRI brain images. A filter for random noise removal was adapted to reduce the noise in MRI images. This parametric filter, named Non-local means, was highly dependent on the setting of its parameters.

Anand et al. [45] discussed a wavelet-based bilateral filtering scheme for noise reduction in magnetic resonance images. In this method, an algorithm was proposed for 2D image de-noising and segmentation using redundant discrete wavelet transform. A two-stage de-noising algorithm was presented for the image segmentation. The importance of noise removal for the MRI was explained.

Cybenko et al. [46] explained the benefit of neural networks that lies in the subsequent theoretical facets. First, the neural networks are data-driven self-adaptive methods in which they can fine-tune themselves to the data exclusive of any clear specification of functional or distributional form for the unique model. Second, they are universal functional approximations in which neural networks can approximate the functions with random accuracy. It explained the importance of classification process in brain tumor detection.

http://dx.doi.org/10.5772/intechopen.71416

Wan et al. [47] reported that the neural networks were non-linear models, which made them stretchable in the model and define real world intricate relationships. The neural networks that are able to approximate the subsequent probabilities, offer the basis for setting up classification rules and statistical analysis.

Pratt et al. [48] explained the RG method that involved the selection of initial seed points. It examined the neighboring pixels as initial "seed points" and determined whether the pixel neighbors should be added to the region or not based on certain conditions. The importance of the seed point selection was also explained.

In all the above methods, region growing methods and it steps for segmenting and detecting tumor in dark abnormalities of the MRI brain images are discussed.

1.4.3. Image segmentation using genetic algorithm-based method

The genetic algorithm (GA) description and some of the recent researches for segmentation based on genetic methodologies are as follows:

The genetic algorithm (GA) is a population-based stochastic search procedure to find exact solutions to the optimization and search problems. The GA creates a sequence of populations for each successive generation by using a selection mechanism and the operators such as selection, crossover, and mutation.

The GA explains an objective function or fitness function value used to evaluate the ability of each chromosome for providing a satisfactory solution to the problem ([49]). The selection procedure, modeled on nature's survival-of-the-fittest mechanism, ensures that the fitter chromosomes have a greater number of off springs in the subsequent generations. For the crossover, two chromosomes are randomly chosen from the population set. After crossover mutation is the second operator which is used for randomizing the search. Mutation alters the content of the chromosomes at a randomly selected position of the chromosome, after determining whether the chromosome satisfies the mutation probability.

Mahindra Pratap Panigrahy et al. [50] proposed a face recognition method using GA and neural networks. The pattern recognition or face recognition problems deal with the combinations of GA with BPNN. The pattern recognition is a problem in time complexity because it requires a careful investigation about different type of patterns for huge database.

Elnomery Zanaty and Ahmed Ghiduk [51] presented a hybridization of the GA and seed region growing to produce medical image segmentation. A new fitness function was presented for generating global minima of the objective function, and a chromosome representation suitable for the process of segmentation was proposed. The RG algorithm used an initial seed point to find accurate regions for each gene. The fitness function was used to evolve the population for getting the best region for each gene. The chromosomes were updated by applying the operators of GA to evolve segmentation results. The time complexity was a drawback of this method, because the calculations of fitness function for each population set took time.

Wang et al. [52] presented a combined GA with clustering FCM method. The parameters in the GA were adjusted adaptively according to the value and the varying velocity of individual fitness to increase the genetic algorithm's adaptability. The constraint based on the second order derivative of histogram was introduced into genetic algorithm to reduce the searching scope and increase the efficiency of calculation. The combined GA with FCM clustering method suffered due to over segmentation problem.

Halder et al. [53] described a GA-based approach for gray-scale image segmentation that segmented the image into various constituent parts automatically. They used FCM clustering to help in generating the population of GA to automatically segment the image. The FCM algorithm assigned pixels to each category by using fuzzy membership function and then adjusted the values of the cluster centers encoded in the chromosome, replacing them by the mean points of the respective clusters. The main disadvantage of the hybridization methods was the difficulty in searching the proper number of classes in case of FCM which lacked the number of clusters.

Mohamad Awad et al. [54] discussed a multi-component image segmentation using a genetic algorithm and artificial neural network. Several methods were developed to segment the multi-component images. The multi component image segmentation method was developed using a non-parametric unsupervised artificial neural network called Kohonen's Self-Organizing Map (SOM) and hybrid genetic algorithm (HGA).The SOM was used to detect the main features of the image; then, HGA is used to cluster the image into homogeneous regions without any prior knowledge. These were performed on different satellite images to confirm the efficiency and robustness of the SOM–HGA method compared with the iterative self-organizing DATA analysis technique (ISODATA).

Peter Angeline et al. [29] stated an evolutionary algorithm that constructed recurrent neural networks. The GA and evolutionary programming are population-based search method that has shown promise in such complex tasks. The standard methods to induct both the structure and weight values of recurrent neural networks have assigned an assumed class of architectures to every task. This paper argued that the GA were inappropriate for the network acquisition and described an evolutionary program that simultaneously acquired both the structure and weights for the recurrent networks.

Insung Jung et al. [55] described a pattern classification of back-propagation algorithm using exclusive connecting network. The objective was to design a pattern classification model for decision support system based on the BP algorithm. The standard BPNN model connected each node from input to output layers. Time complexity of the algorithm was high and the error rate was small when the training was performed.

Amiya Halder et al. [56] proposed an unsupervised dynamic image segmentation using fuzzy Hopfield neural network with genetic algorithm. The genetic algorithm-based segmentation method could automatically segment the gray-scale images. This method mainly explained the spatial unsupervised gray-scale image segmentation that divided an image into regions. The aim of this algorithm was to produce a precise segmentation of images using intensity information along with neighborhood relationships. Fuzzy Hopfield Neural Network (FHNN) clustering helps to generate the population of genetic algorithm and it automatically segments the images with good quality.

Maulik [57] presented a detailed survey of the applications of GAs to medical image segmentation. The main challenges and issues in integrating GA for solving the optimization problems in medical image segmentation were presented. The choices of the different genetic operators as well as the termination criteria were discussed. The important issues in GA and the expert knowledge, integration with local search algorithms were also discussed.

David Montana et al. [58] proposed training feed forward neural networks using genetic algorithms. The multilayered feed forward neural networks possess a number of properties which make them particularly suited to complex pattern classification problems. The genetic algorithms are a class of optimization procedures which are good at exploring a large and complex space in an intelligent way to find the values close to the global optimum. Hence, they are well suited to the problem of training feed forward networks.

1.5. Results and discussion

This section describes some of the experimental results of the proposed GFSMRG with BPNN technique using the MRI brain images with and without tumor. The preprocessed image and histogram generated image are shown in **Figure 12**.

1.6. Conclusion

MRI using segmentation method is an important diagnostic tool for the prediction of brain tumors. This chapter explains about the different segmentation methodologies for brain tumor segmentation. With a sound mechanism and clear imaging of soft tissues, the diagnosis of a patient can be scientific and rational segmentation can do with new artificial methodologies. It enables the doctors to grasp the exact progression of the disease state, which would help to make a decision about the appropriate treatment, surgery and following-up for a series of disease control measures. The computer-aided and automated segmentation tool and its analysis has reduced the workload of doctors and improved the diagnostic accuracy of the paramedical analysis.

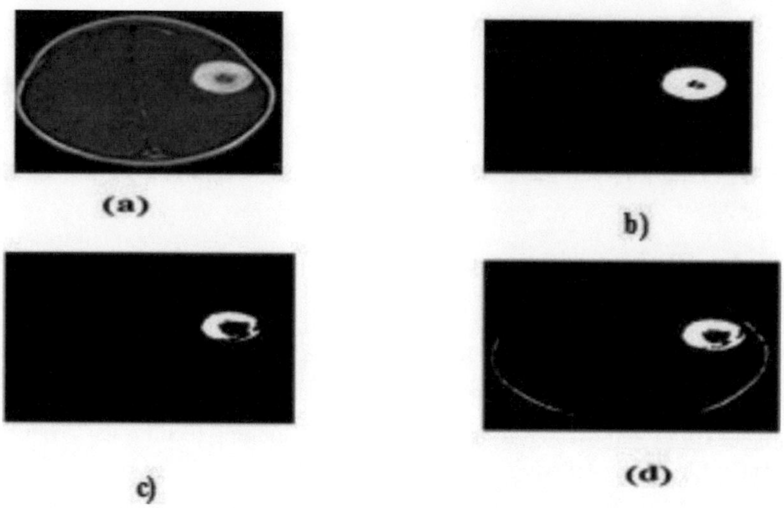

Figure 12. (a) Input image, (b) FCM [21], (c) RG (Shafaf [31]), and (d) GA with fuzzy ([59].

Author details

Kavitha Angamuthu Rajasekaran* and Chellamuthu Chinna Gounder

*Address all correspondence to: arkavithabalaji@gmail.com

Anna University, Chennai, Tamil Nadu, India

References

[1] Falk T, Shatkay H, Chan WY. Breast Cancer Prognosis via Gaussian Mixture regression. Proceedings of Canadian Conference on Electrical and Computer Eng. (CCECE '06). 2006;**64**(1):987-990

[2] Fan Y, Rao H, Giannetta J, Hurt H, Wang J, Davatzikos C, Shen D. Diagnosis of brain abnormality using both structural and functional MR images. Conference on Proceedings of IEEE Engineering Medical and Biology Society. 2006;**11**(8):1044-1047

[3] Gonzalez RC. Digital Image Processing. Peking: Publishing House of Electronics Industry; 2003

[4] Shen D, Herskovits E, Davatzikos C. An adaptative-focus statistical shape model for segmentation and shape modeling of 3D brain structures. IEEE Transaction on Medical Imaging. 2001;**3**(4):257-270

[5] Li S, Tan M. Gene selection and tissue classification based on support vector machine and genetic algorithm. IEEE International Conference on Bio-Informatics and Biomedical Engineering. 2007;**7**(4):244-259

[6] Stark DD, Bradley WG. Magnetic Resonance Imaging. 3rd ed. Mosby; 1999. pp. 1321-1254

[7] Steen RG. Edema and tumor perfusion: Characterization by quantitative HMR imaging. American Journal of Radiology. 1992;**158**:259-264

[8] Huang JY, Liang XY. The Basic Principles of Medical Imaging. Beijing: Electronic Industry Press; 2009

[9] Zhan Y, Tan GX. Medical Imaging Diagnostic Lab Manual. Wuhan Hubei Science and Technology Press; 2009

[10] Yang ZH, Feng F, Wang XY. MRI guide-check specification, clinical strategies and application of new technologies. Beijing: People's Medical Publishing House. 2010;**5**(2):34-49

[11] Armstrong TS, Cohen MZ, Weinbrg J, Gilbert MR. Imaging techniques in neuro oncology. Seminars in Oncology Nursing. 2004;**20**(4):231-239

[12] Jacobs MA, Ibrahim TS, Ouwerkerk R. MR imaging: Brief overview and emerging applications. Radio Graphics. 2007;**27**(4):1213-1229

[13] Haacke M, Brown R, Thompson M, Venkatesan R. Magnetic Resonance Imaging: Physical Principles and Sequence Design. New York: Wiley-Liss; 1999

[14] Bushberg J, Seibert A, Leidholdt E, Boone J. Essential Physics of Medical Imaging. Philadelphia: Lippincott Williams & Wilkins; 2002;**10**(2):1335-1347

[15] Cruickshank G. Tumours of the brain surgery. Oxford. 2004;**22**(3):69-72

[16] www.usa.siemens.com/healthcare, 2012

[17] Wu EH, Feng GS, Bai RJ. Medical imaging (the 6th edition). Beijing: People's Medical Publishing House, vol. 40, no. 9, pp. 156-163

[18] Tsuchiya K, Mizutani Y, Hachiya J. Preliminary evaluation of fluid attenuated inversion-recovery MR in the diagnosis of intracranial tumors. American Journal of Neuro radiology. 1996;**17**(6):1081-1086

[19] Wang CZ. Neurosurgery. Beijing: People's Medical Publishing House. 2002;**47**(12):456-459

[20] Seer 2011, www.abta.org

[21] Jude Hemanth D, Selvathi D, Anitha J. Effective Fuzzy Clustering Algorithm for Abnormal MR Brain Image Segmentation. International Advance Computing Conference. 2009;**13**(7):609-614

[22] Kaiqi Z, Zhiping W, Ming H. An Improved FCM algorithm for Color Image Segmentation. The 3rd International Conference on Innovative Computing Information and Control (ICICIC'08). 2009;**22**(4):15-27

[23] Pham DL, Xu CY, Prince JL. A survey of current methods in medical image segmentation. Annual Review of Biomedical Engineering. 2008;**2**(7):315-337

[24] HemaRajini N, Bhavani R. Enhancing K-means and Kernelized fuzzy C-means clustering with cluster center initialization in segmenting MRI brain images. IEEE 3rd International Conference on Electronics Computer Technology (ICECT). 2011;**2**(7):259-263

[25] Caldairou B, Passat N, Habas PA, Studholme C, Rousseau F. A non-local fuzzy segmentation method: Application to brain MRI. Pattern Recognition. 2011;**44**(9):1916-1927

[26] Kim Y, Kang M, Kim J-M. Exploration of Optimal Many-Core Models for Efficient Image Segmentation. IEEE Transactions on Image Processing. 2013;**22**(6):1767-1777

[27] Sandham W. 'MRI fuzzy segmentation of brain tissue using neighborhood attraction with neural-network optimization', IEEE Transactions on Information Technology in Biomedicine, 2005;**9**(3):67-78

[28] Gong M, Liang Y, Shi J, Ma W, Ma J. Fuzzy C-means clustering with local information and kernel metric for image segmentation. IEEE transactions on. Image processing. 2013;**22**(2):573-584

[29] Angeline PJ, Saunders GM, Pollack JB. An evolutionary algorithm that constructs recurrent neural networks. International Journal of Computer Science. 1995;**23**(4):88-97

[30] Zulaikha Beevi S, Mohamed Sathik M. An effective approach for segmentation of MRI images: Combining spatial information with fuzzy C-means clustering. European Journal of Scientific Research. 2010;**41**(3):437-451

[31] Ibrahim S, Khalid NEA, Manaf M. Seed-based region growing (SBRG) vs adaptive network-based inference system (ANFIS) vs fuzzy c-means (FCM): Brain abnormalities segmentation. International Journal of Electrical and Computer Engineering. 2010;**5**(2):94-104

[32] Zhu L, Gao Y, Yezzi A, Tannenbaum A. Automatic Segmentation of the Left Atrium from MR Images via Variation Region Growing With a Moments-Based Shape Prior. IEEE Transactions on Image Processing. 2013;**22**(7):1057-1071

[33] Cai Y, Baciu G. Detecting, Grouping, and Structure Inference for Invariant Repetitive Patterns in Images. IEEE Transactions on. image processing. 2013;**22**(7):2343-2355

[34] Nigri Happ P, Queiroz Feitosa R, Bentes C, Farias R. A region growing segmentation algorithm for GPUs. IEEE Geosciences and Remote Sensing Letters. 2013;**10**(30):1612-1616

[35] Kaushik AC, Sharma V. Brain tumor segmentation from MRI images and volume calculation of tumor. International Journal of Pharmaceutical Science Invention. 2013;**7**(2):23-26

[36] Bhoi N, Meher S. Total variation based wavelet domain filter for image denoising. Proc. 1st Int. Conf. on Emerging trends in engineering and technology: ICETET 08, Nagpur, India, July, G. H. Raisoni College of Engineering. 2008;**3**(3):20-25

[37] Bhandarkar SM, Nammalwar P. Segmentation of multispectral MR images using a hierarchical self-organizing map. Proc. 14th IEEE Symp. On Computer based medical system. CBMS Bethesda, MD, USA: IEEE Computer Society. 2001;**6**(6);294-299

[38] Tilton J. Analysis of hierarchically related image segmentations. IEEE workshop on advances in technique for analysis of remotely sensed data. 2003;**8**(8):123-139

[39] Jabbar NI, Mehrotra M. Application of fuzzy neural network for image tumor description. Proceeding of World Acadamy of Science Engineering Technology. 2008;**2**(8):427-429

[40] Jaya J, Thanushkodi K, Karnan M. Tracking algorithm for de-noising of MR brain images. IJCSNS Int. J. Comput. Sci. Network Secur. 2009;**9**(11):262-267

[41] Wu J, Albert CS , Chung. 'A novel framework for segmentation of deep brain structures based on Markov dependence tree', NeuroImage. 2009;**46**(8):1027-1036

[42] Kekre HB, Sarode T, Raut K. Detection of tumor in MRI using vector quantization segmentation. International Journal of Computer Application. 2010;**4**(9):14-19

[43] Corso JJ, Sharon E, Dube S, El-Saden S, Sinha U, Yuilles A. Efficient multilevel brain tumor segmentation with integrated Bayesian model classification. IEEE Transactions on Medical Imaging. 2008;**27**(15):629-640

[44] Liao L, Lin TS, Li B. MRI brain image segmentation and bias field correction based on fast spatially constrained kernel clustering approach. Journal of Pattern Recognition Letters. 2008;**29**(5):1580-1588

[45] Anand CS, Sahambi JS. Wavelet domain nonlinear filtering for MRI denoising. Magnetic Resonance Imaging. 2010;**28**(6):842-861

[46] Cybenko L, Fan C. Robust classification for extraction for magnetic resonance imaging. IEEE Geoscience and Remote Sensing Letters. 1991;**5**(2):246-250

[47] Wan E. Neural network classification: A Bayesian interpretation. IEEE Transactions on Neural Networks. 1990;**1**(1):303-313

[48] Pratt WK. Digital Image Processing. 4th ed. Los Altos, CA: John Wiley & Sons, Inc.; 2007

[49] Holland JH. Adaptation in Neural and Artificial Systems. University of Michigan press; 1975

[50] Panigrahy MP, Kumar N. Face recognition using genetic algorithm and neural networks. International Journal of Computer Applications. 2012;**55**(4):145-157

[51] ElnomeryZanaty A, Ahmed Ghiduk S. A novel approach based on genetic algorithms and region growing for magnetic resonance image (MRI) segmentation. ComSIS. 2013; **10**(3):1319-1342

[52] Wang H, Zhang BJ, Liu XZ, Luo DZ, Zhong SB. Image segmentation method based on improved genetic algorithm and fuzzy clustering. Advanced Materials Research. 2011;**379**(7):143-144

[53] Halder A, Pramanik S, Karm A. Dynamic image segmentation using fuzzy CMeans based genetic algorithm. International Journal of Computer Applications. 2011;**28**(6):15-20

[54] Awad M, Chehdi K, Nasri A. 'Multicomponent image segmentation using a genetic algorithm and artificial neural network', IEEE Geoscience and Remote Sensing Letters. 2007;**4**(4):571-575

[55] Jung I, Wang G-N. Pattern classification of back-propagation algorithm using exclusive connecting network. World Academy of Science, Engineering and Technology. 2007;**36**(6): 180-184

[56] Halder A, Pramanik S. An unsupervised dynamic image segmentation using fuzzy Hopfield neural network based genetic algorithm. IJCSI International Journal of Computer Science. 2012;**9**(2):525-532

[57] Maulik U. 'Medical image segmentation using genetic algorithms', IEEE Transactions on Information Technology in Biomedicine. 2009;**13**(2):166-173

[58] David Montana J, Davis L. Training feedforward neural networks using genetic algorithms. MachineLearning. 2008;**1**(89):762-767

[59] Kaur A, Jindal G. Tumour detection using genetic algorithm. International Journal of Computer Science And Technology. 2013;**4**(1):423-427

Section 2

Physical Sciences, Engineering and Technology

Chapter 7

MRI Medical Image Denoising by Fundamental Filters

Hanafy M. Ali

Additional information is available at the end of the chapter

http://dx.doi.org/10.5772/intechopen.72427

Abstract

Nowadays Medical imaging technique Magnetic Resonance Imaging (MRI) plays an important role in medical setting to form high standard images contained in the human brain. MRI is commonly used once treating brain, prostate cancers, ankle and foot. The Magnetic Resonance Imaging (MRI) images are usually liable to suffer from noises such as Gaussian noise, salt and pepper noise and speckle noise. So getting of brain image with accuracy is very extremely task. An accurate brain image is very necessary for further diagnosis process. During this chapter, a median filter algorithm will be modified. Gaussian noise and Salt and pepper noise will be added to MRI image. A proposed Median filter (MF), Adaptive Median filter (AMF) and Adaptive Wiener filter (AWF) will be implemented. The filters will be used to remove the additive noises present in the MRI images. The noise density will be added gradually to MRI image to compare performance of the filters evaluation. The performance of these filters will be compared exploitation the applied mathematics parameter Peak Signal-to-Noise Ratio (PSNR).

Keywords: MRI image, de-noising, non-linear filter, median filter, adaptive filter and, adaptive median filter

1. Introduction

Statistical models of signal and noise consider a fundamental role in medical image processing. In particular, many different applications in the magnetic resonance (MR) image processing field rely on a well-defined prior statistical model of the data. Many techniques of these model-based methods may be found in literature: noise removal and signal estimation methods as the conventional approach.

MR image De-noising has been an important research point in the field of MR image processing. Noise reduction and removing process is an important part of MR image processing systems. It is a technique removes out noise which is added in the MR original image. MR Image quality may get defective while capturing, processing and storing the MR image. Removing noise from the original MR images is still a challenging problem for researchers because noise removal introduces artifacts and causes blurring of the MR images. Nowadays, MR image de-noising has become an important purpose in medical imaging particularly the Magnetic Resonance Imaging (MRI). Many de-noising and enhancement techniques are applied on MRI images [1–8].

De-noising is one of the main branches of MR image processing. Basically, it finds its major use in all of the systems that acquire mono-dimensional or multi-dimensional signals. Of course, Magnetic Resonance Imaging (MRI), which plays an important role in clinical diagnosis producing high quality 2-D and 3-D images of the body, is also affected by noise. Several de-noising techniques have been proposed in recent years in literature. The main challenge consists in reducing the amount of noise, i.e. regularize the MR image, while preserving the details, the edges and in general the small structures that could be crucial for a correct diagnosis. Three main MRI de-noising filter families can be identified: methods defined in the spatial domain, methods working in a transformed domain and methods exploiting the statistical properties of the signals. Filters in the spatial domain implement an average of pixels for reducing the amount of noise.

In this chapter, a median filter algorithm will be modified. Gaussian noise and Salt and pepper noise will be added to MRI image. A proposed Median filter (MF), Adaptive Median filter (AMF) and Adaptive Wiener filter (AWF) will be implemented. The filters will be used to remove the additive noises present in the MRI images. The noise density will be added gradually to MRI image to compare performance of the filters evaluation. The performance of these filters will be compared exploitation the applied mathematics parameter Peak Signal-to-Noise Ratio (PSNR). After this study, the best filtering method for MRI image will be able to define.

2. Image denoising techniques

A lot of different MR image de-noising techniques are developed so far each having its own advantages and limitation. According this work will prove that, applied the technique depend on the type and amount of noise present in the MR image. One should also consider the other factors like performance in de-noising the MR image, computational time, and computational cost [9–12].

De-noising can be exhausted in various domains like Spatial Domain, Frequency Domain and Wavelet Domain. Also, filtering is a technique in MR image processing which is employed for various tasks like noise reduction, interpolation, and re-sampling. The selection of filter depends upon the type and amount of noise present in an image because different filters can remove different types of noise efficiently.

2.1. Adaptive Wiener filter

Adaptive Wiener Filter (AWF) is considering frequency domain filter. The adaptive Wiener filter changes its behavior based on the statistical characteristics of the MR image inside the filter region, which is defined by the maximum rectangular window. Adaptive filter performance is commonly superior to non-adaptive counterparts. Mean and variance are two important mathematics measures using which adaptive filters can be designed [13].

The adaptive Wiener filter uses a pixel-wise adaptive Wiener method based on statistics estimated from a local neighborhood of each pixel. Its function filters the MR image using pixel-wise adaptive Wiener filtering, using neighborhoods of size M-by-N to estimate the local MR image mean and standard deviation.

2.2. Non-linear filters

In recent years, a variety of non-linear filters like median filter, adaptive median filter, min filter, max filter have been developed to overcome the defect of linear filter. Non-linear filters give better performance than linear filters [12, 14]. The non-linear filters are spatial domain filters. In following sections, the median filter and adaptive median filter are discussed.

2.2.1. The proposal median filter

Median filter is spatial domain filter. It is also define as order statistics filter. The median filter is most common and commonly used nonlinear filter. It removes noise by smoothing the MR images. This filter also lowers the intensity variation between one and other pixels of an MR image. The median filter algorithm replaced the pixel value of MR image with the median value. The median value is calculated in two steps, first step; arranging all the pixel values in ascending order, second step; replace the pixel being calculated with the middle pixel value. If the neighboring pixel of MR image which is to be consider, contains and even no of pixels, then it replaces the pixel with average of two middle pixel values. The mean filter can be represented by the following equation:

$$f^{\wedge}(x, y) = \text{median}\{g(s, t)\} \quad \text{where } (s, t) \in S_{xy} \tag{1}$$

where S_{xy} is corresponds to the set of coordinates in a rectangular sub MR image window which has center at (x, y). The median filter calculates the median of the corrupted MR image g(x,y) under the area S_{xy}. Here f^(x, y) represents the restored MR image.

In this chapter, the median filter algorithm is modified. The restored MR image pixel at (i,j) equal the median value of (g(i−1, j), g(i, j−1), g(i + 1, j), g(i, j + 1), g(i + 1, j + 1), g(i−1, j−1), g(i−1,j + 1) and g(i + 1, j−1).

Median filters are mostly used by researchers due to its capability to fit out excellent noise reduction with less blurring for various types of noise. Median filters are wide used as smoothers for MR image processing, as well as in signal processing and time series processing. A major advantage of the median filter over linear filters is that the median filter can eliminate and remove the effect of input noise values with extremely large magnitudes.

2.2.2. Adaptive median filtering

The Adaptive Median Filtering (AMF) [15] has been applied wide as an advanced de-noising technique compared with traditional median filtering. The adaptive Median filter executes spatial processing to determine which pixels in an MR image have been affected by noise. The Adaptive Median Filter classifies pixels as noise by comparison each pixel in the MR image to its surrounding neighbor pixels. The size of the neighborhood window is adjustable, as well as the threshold for the comparison. A pixel that is different from a majority of its neighbors, as well as being not structurally aligned with those pixels to which it is similar, is labeled as noisy pixel. These noisy pixels are then exchange by the median value of the pixels in the neighborhood that have passed the noise labeling test. Adaptive median filter changes the size of the neighborhood window through operation. But, in classic median filter; the neighborhood window is constant through the operation. For that, the standard median filter does not perform well when the impulse noise density is high, while the adaptive median filter can better handle these noises. Also, the adaptive median filter preserves MR image details such as edges and smooth non-impulsive noise, while the standard median filter does not.

In this chapter, the adaptive median filter works on a rectangular region S_{xy}. The adaptive median filter changes the size of S_{xy} through the filtering operation depending on certain criteria. The adaptive median filter works in two levels denoted Level A and Level B as follows.

Level 1: $L_{11} = Z_{med} - Z_{min}$

$L12 = Z_{med} - Z_{max}$

If $L_{11} > 0$ AND $L_{12} < 0$, Go to level 2

Else increase the window size.

If window size <= S_{max} repeat level 1.

Else output Z_{xy}.

Level 2: $L_{21} = Z_{xy} - Z_{min}$

$L22 = Z_{xy} - Z_{min}$

If $L_{21} > 0$ And $L_{22} < 0$ output Z_{xy}

Else output Z_{med}.

Where

Z_{min} is a minimum gray level value in S_{xy}.

Z_{max} is a maximum gray level value in S_{xy}.

Z_{med} is a median of gray levels in S_{xy}.

Z_{xy} is a gray level at coordinates (x, y).

S_{max} is a maximum allowed size of $_{Sxy}$.

The output of the filter is a single value which the exchange the corrupted pixel MR image value at (x, y), the point on which S_{xy} is centered at the time.

3. Common noises in MR image

From theoretical expectations, the noise measured in unfiltered MR images was found to be usually distributed, spatially invariant and white. As in MR image processing, the MR images are much sensitive to noise which results are due to the image acquisition errors and transmission errors. MR images captured usually are prone to Gaussian noise and salt and pepper noise which has influence on the MR image quality [4, 16–22]. Poor quality of MR image tends to degrade the performances of any works such as feature extraction, reduction and classification of the processed MR images. The noises go to be removed before these processing stages as there were many available MR image filtering algorithms recommended in the literature. Gaussian noise and Impulse noise are popular noises distributed in magnitude MR images and non-avoidable. Because of its mathematical tractability in both the spatial and frequency domains, many of filters are used to remove the Gaussian noise. Salt and pepper noise consider as impulsive noise will have dark pixels and bright pixels alternate bright and dark regions. Because impulse corruption usually is large compared with the strength of the image signal, the impulse noise mostly is digitized as extreme values in an image.

3.1. Gaussian noise or amplifier noise

It is conjointly referred to as Gaussian distribution. The Gaussian noise has a probability density equation of the normal distribution. The Gaussian noise or amplifier noise is added to MR image during image acquisition such as sensor noise caused by low light, high temperature, transmission e.g. electronic circuit noise. This noise will be removed by using spatial filtering (Adaptive Wiener filter, Median filter, Wiener filter and Adaptive Median filter). The Probabilities Density Function (PDF) of Gaussian Noise is shown in the following equation and **Figure 1**:

$$p(z) = \frac{1}{\sqrt{2\pi\sigma}} e^{\frac{-(z-u)^2}{2\sigma^2}} \quad (2)$$

where $P_{(x)}$ is the Gaussian distribution equation noise in MR image; μ and σ is the mean and standard deviation respectively.

3.2. Impulse noise

The Impulse noise is also defined by Salt & Pepper noise or Spike noise. It is caused by malfunctioning pixels in camera sensors, faulty memory locations in hardware, or transmission

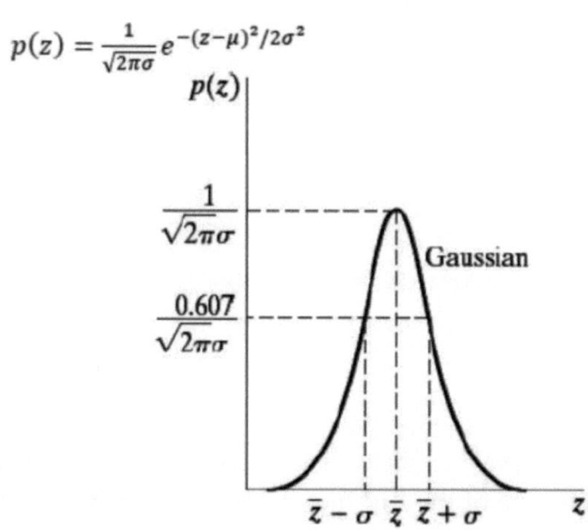

Figure 1. Gaussian noise.

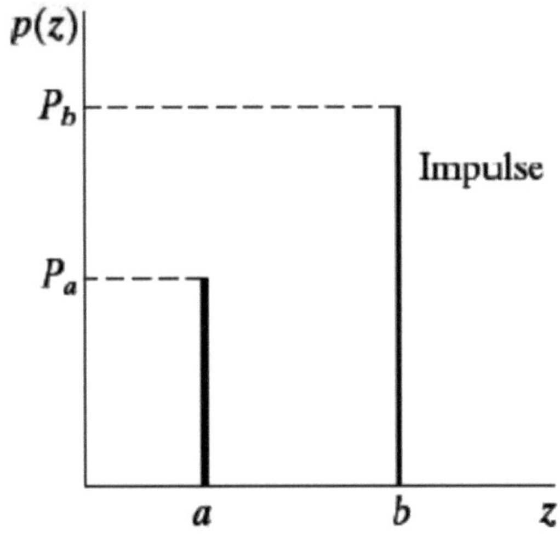

Figure 2. Salt and pepper noise.

in a noisy channel. It is forever independent and uncorrelated to MR image pixels. Its two types are the salt-and-pepper noise and the random-valued noise. In the Salt and Pepper type of noise, the noisy pixels takes either salt value (gray level – 225) or pepper value (gray level – 0) and it seems as black and white spots on the MR images In case of random valued impulse noise, noise can take any gray level value from 0 to 225. In this case also noise is randomly distributed over the entire MR image and probability of occurrence of any gray level value as noise will be same. The Salt and Pepper noise is shown in following equation and **Figure 2**.

$$P(z) = \begin{cases} P_a & \text{for } z = a \\ P_b & \text{for } z = b \\ 0 & \text{otherwise} \end{cases} \tag{3}$$

where p_a, p_b are the probabilities density equation, p (z) is distribution salt and pepper noise in MR image and a, b are the arrays size MR image.

4. Peak signal-to-noise ratio

The phrase peak signal-to-noise ratio is typically abbreviated PSNR. The peak signal-to-noise ratio (PSNR) is an engineering term defined as the ratio between the maximum possible power of a signal and the power of corrupting noise that affects the fidelity of its representation. Because many signals have a very wide dynamic range, PSNR is typically expressed in terms of the logarithmic decibel scale.

It is most simply defined via the mean squared error (MSE) which for two m × n monochrome MR images I and K where one of the MR images is considered a noisy approximation of the other is defined as:

$$\text{MSE} = \frac{1}{mn}\sum_{i=0}^{m-1}\sum_{j=0}^{n-1}[I(i,j) - K(i,j)]^2 \quad (4)$$

The PSNR equation is defined as:

$$\text{PSNR} = 20.\log_{10}\left(\frac{\text{MAX}}{\sqrt{\text{MSE}}}\right) = 10.\log_{10}\left(\frac{\text{MAX}^2}{\text{MSE}}\right) \quad (5)$$

Here, MAX is the maximum possible pixel value of the MR image. When the pixels are represented using 8 bits per sample, this is 255. More generally, when samples are represented using linear PCM with B bits per sample, MAX is $2^B - 1$.

5. Results and discussion

The three filters: the adaptive Wiener filter, the median filter and the adaptive median filter were implemented using (MATLAB R22015a) and tested for two types of noise: Gaussian Noise and Salt & Pepper Noise corrupted on the MRI brain image. The following two sections describe the results.

5.1. Qualitative analysis

Figures 3(A)–(C) and **8(A)–(B)** present MRI image with different noise density (10%, 50% and 90%). The quality of image is rebuilding using Adaptive Wiener, Median and Adaptive Median filters. The Adaptive Wiener filter result is showed bad filter MRI image quality for Salt and Pepper and Gaussian noise. The results of the Median filter showed, its better filter

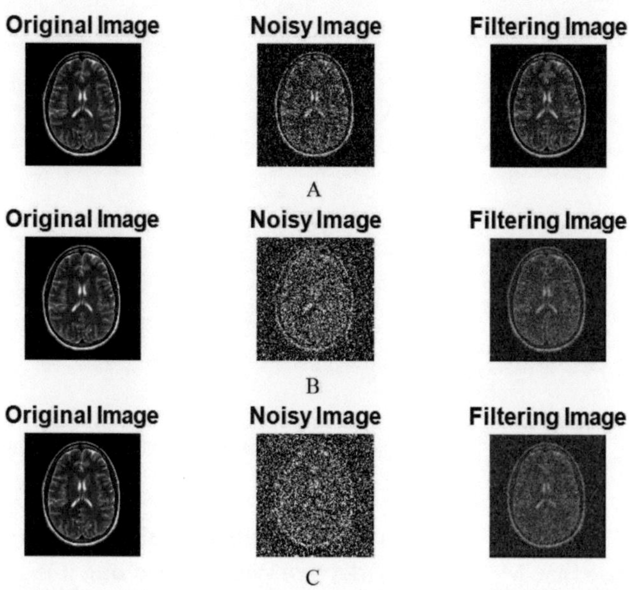

Figure 3. Wiener filter (Gaussian noise). (A) Noise Density =10%- PSNR=43.2096, (B) Noise Density =50%- PSNR=37.9244, (C) Noise Density =90%- PSNR=36.5301.

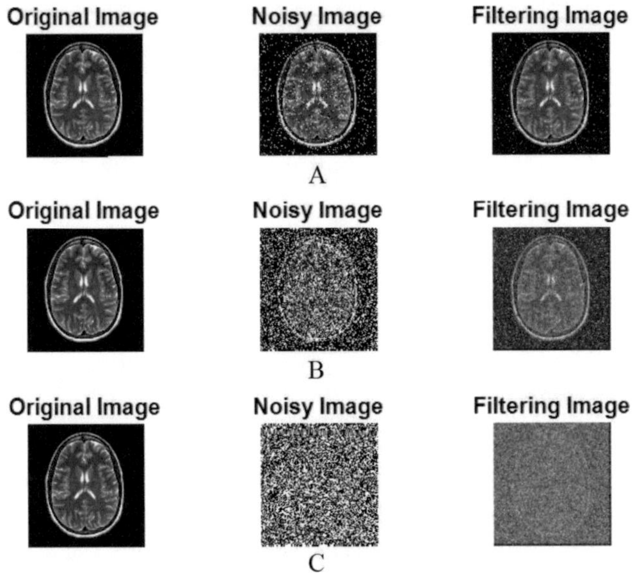

Figure 4. Wiener filter (Salt & Pepper Noise). (A) Noise Density =10%- PSNR=45.2549, (B) Noise Density =50%- PSNR=37.8006, (C) Noise Density =90%- PSNR=33.4716.

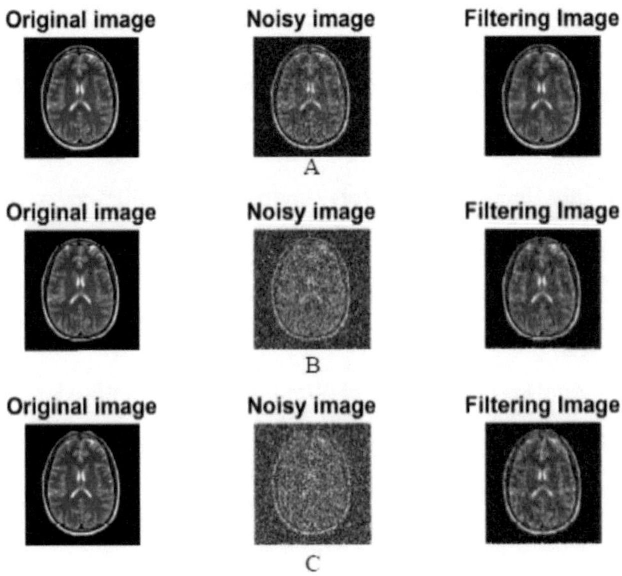

Figure 5. Median filter (Gaussian noise). (A) Noise Density =10%- PSNR=51.9813, (B) Noise Density =50%- PSNR=47.2688, (C) Noise Density =90%- PSNR=45.5434.

image quality for Gaussian noise. The Adaptive Median results showed, it is better filter for salt and Pepper noise than Median and Adaptive Wiener filter. But, it is gave bad filter quality for Gaussian noise. The PSNR is recorded below for each resultant image as shown in **Figures 3–8**. In this work, the calculation algorithm of median value in median filter is modified. The processing time and memory used for median filter algorithm was increase than the Adaptive Wiener and Adaptive Median filters by 400%.

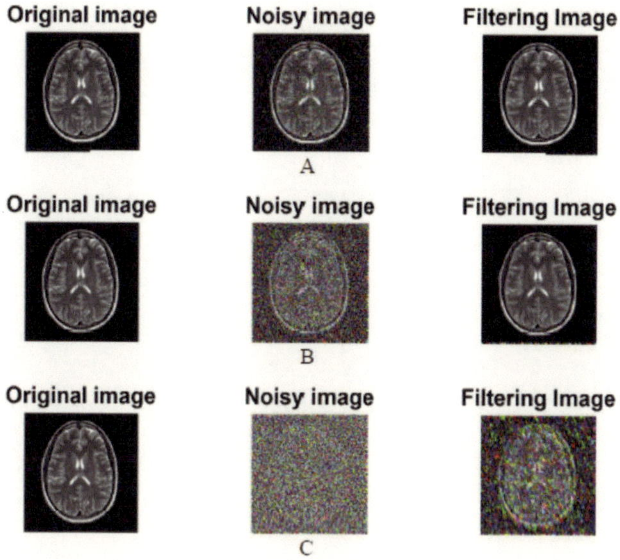

Figure 6. Median filter (Salt & Pepper Noise). (A) Noise Density =10%- PSNR=61.8162, (B) Noise Density =50%- PSNR=52.0523, (C) Noise Density =90%- PSNR=39.1255.

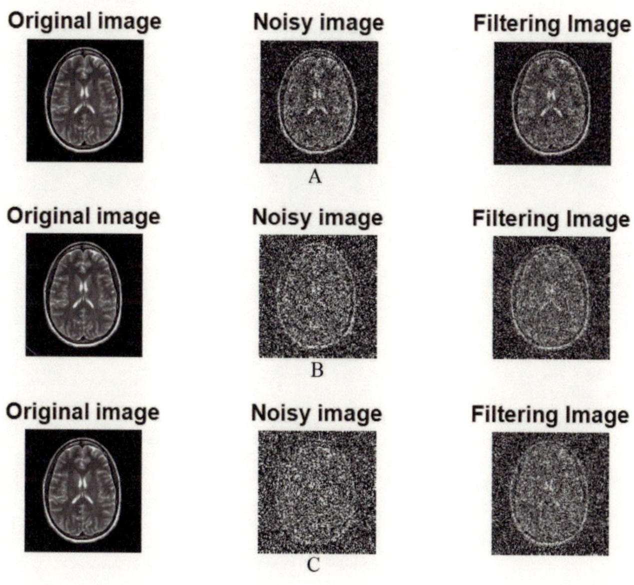

Figure 7. Adaptive median filter (Gaussian noise). (A) Noise Density =10%- PSNR=38.9811, (B) Noise Density =50%- PSNR=34.5541, (C) Noise Density =90%- PSNR=33.7908.

5.2. Quantitative analysis

Table 1 shows average peak signal-to-noise ratio (PSNR) values of each tested filters (Adaptive Wiener filter, Median filter and Adaptive Median filter). Each filter was used to remove the Gaussian noise. The noise density was added to MRI image varying from a 10–90%. To compare all three filters, Median filter works better for Gaussian noise as shown in **Figure 9**.

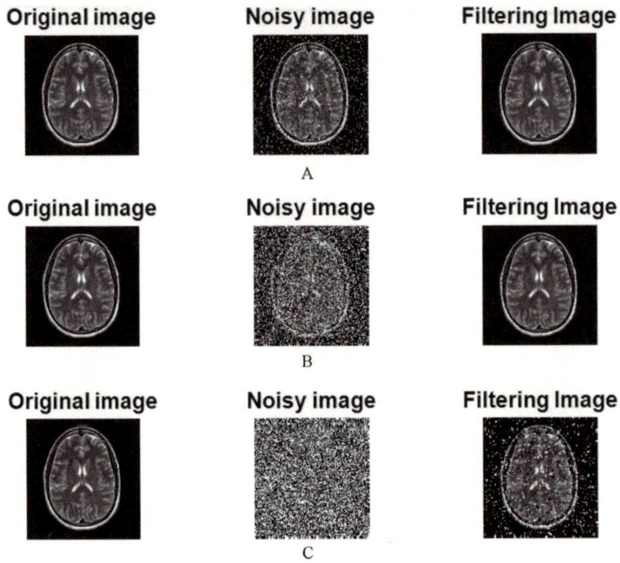

Figure 8. Adaptive median filter (Salt & Pepper Noise). (A) Noise Density =10%- PSNR=66.8579, (B) Noise Density =50%- PSNR=54.9245, (C) Noise Density =90%- PSNR=40.1885.

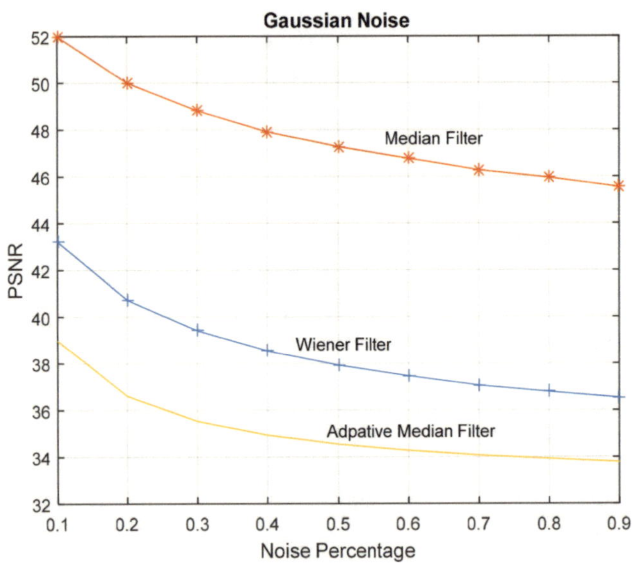

Figure 9. PSNR of different filtering methods (Gaussian noise).

Median filter performs higher PSNR compared to other filters as shown in **Table 1**. Also, the efficiency of Adaptive Median filter is bad in removing Gaussian noise and more blurring occurs in the image as shown in **Figure 7** and **Table 1**.

Gaussian Noise	10%	20%	30%	40%	50%	60%	70%	80%	90%
Wiener	43.2096	40.7198	39.4058	38.5437	37.9244	37.4609	37.0554	36.7821	36.5301
Median	51.9813	50.0028	48.8096	47.9059	47.2688	46.7664	46.2666	45.9440	45.5434
Adaptive median	38.9811	36.6111	35.5311	34.9378	34.5541	34.2792	34.0766	33.9278	33.7908

Table 1. PSNR of different filtering methods (Gaussian noise).

Salt & Pepper Noise	10%	20%	30%	40%	50%	60%	70%	80%	90%
Wiener	45.2549	42.7827	40.8778	39.2039	37.8006	36.5460	35.3685	34.3821	33.4716
Median	61.8162	58.7794	56.6603	54.2224	52.0523	49.3339	46.5512	43.2658	39.1255
Adaptive median	66.8579	62.3232	59.4506	57.2552	54.9245	52.8025	50.6639	45.7517	40.1885

Table 2. PSNR of different filtering methods (Salt & Pepper Noise).

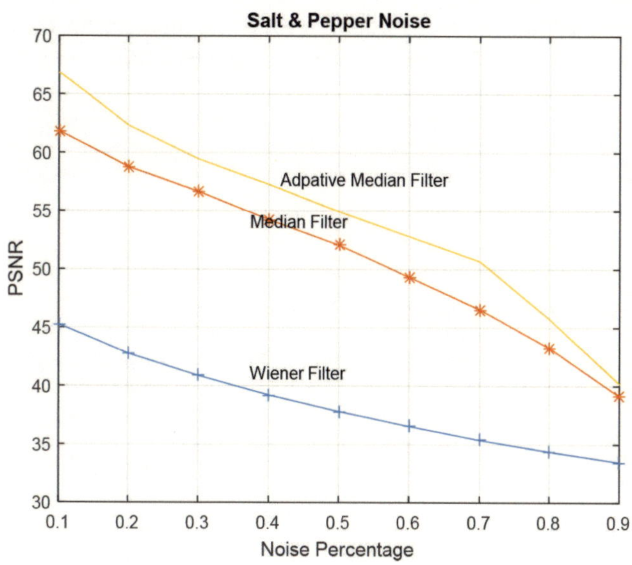

Figure 10. PSNR of different filtering methods (Salt & Pepper Noise).

Table 2 tabulates average peak signal-to-noise ratio (PSNR) values of each tested filters (Adaptive Wiener filter, Median filter and Adaptive Median filter). Each filter was used to take off the Salt and Pepper noise. The noise density was added to MRI image varying from a 10–90%. To compare all three filters, the Adaptive Median filter gave a better result as shown in **Figure 10** and **Table 2**. The Adaptive Median filter performs higher PSNR compared to the Median filter and the Adaptive Weiner filter.

Through this work, the Median filter allowed a high performance in removing two noises (salt and Pepper noise- Gaussian noise). But, the processing time and memory for median filter algorithm was increased than the Adaptive Wiener and Adaptive Median filters by 400%.

6. Conclusion

This paper investigated the performance of three different completely filtering methods tested with different noises on Magnetic Resonance Imaging (MRI) images. The Median filter is the most high performance method as compared to other filters mainly for Gaussian noise de-noising. The Adaptive Median filter is the most outperformed method as compared to other filters mainly for Salt and Pepper noise de-noising.

Through this work proved, the choice of filter depends upon the type and amount of noise present in an image. Also, the de-noising the MRI images performance depends on the type of noise and type of filtering techniques. The Median filter was better filter Magnetic Resonance Imaging images quality Gaussian noise. The Adaptive Median filter was better filter MRI image quality Salt and Pepper noise. The results showed that The Median filter has a better performance than other filters. The computation time and memory for the Median filter algorithm was increased than the Adaptive Wiener and Adaptive Median filters by 400%.

Author details

Hanafy M. Ali

Address all correspondence to: hmali@mu.edu.eg

Computers and Systems Engineering Department, Faculty of Engineering, Minia University, El Minia, Egypt

References

[1] Rajeesh J, Moni RS, Palanikumar S, Gopalakrishnan T. Noise reduction in magnetic resonance images using wave atom shrinkage. International Journal of Image Processing (IJIP). 2010;**4**(2):131-141

[2] Zhang M, Gunturk BK. Multi resolution bilateral filtering for image de-noising. IEEE Transactions on Image Processing. 2008;**17**(12):2324-2333

[3] Phophalia A, Rajwade A, Mitra SK. Rough set based image de-noising for brain MR images. Signal Processing. 2014;**103**(2014):24-35

[4] Isa IS, Sulaiman SN, Mustapha M, Darus S. Evaluating de-noising performances of fundamental filters for T2-weighted MRI images. 19th International Conference on Knowledge Based and Intelligent Information and Engineering Systems. Procedia Computer Science. 2015;**60**:760-768

[5] Rahmat R, Malik AS, Kamel N. Comparison of LULU and median filter for image de-noising. International Journal of Computer and Electrical Engineering. 2013;**5**(6)

[6] Dey N, Ashour AS, Beagum S, Sifaki Pistola D, Gospodinov M, Gospodinova E, Tavares RS. Parameter optimization for local polynomial approximation based intersection confidence interval filter using genetic algorithm: An application for brain MRI image de-noising. Journal of Imaging. 2015;**1**(1):60-84 www.mdpi.com/journal/jimaging

[7] Lakshmi Devasena C, Hemalatha M. Noise removal in magnetic resonance images using hybrid KSL filtering technique. International Journal of Computer Applications (0975-8887);**27**(8):2011

[8] Akar SA. Determination of optimal parameters for bilateral filter in brain MRimage denoising. Applied Soft Computing. 2016;**43**:87-96

[9] Bovik A. Handbook of Image and Video Processing. New York: Academic; 2000

[10] Bourne R. Image filters. In: Fundamentals of Digital Imaging in Medicine. Springer London; 2010

[11] Patel K, Mewada H. A review on different image de-noising methods. International Journal on Recent and Innovation Trends in Computing and Communication. 2014;**2**(1): 155-159

[12] Erturk M. De-noising MRI using spectral subtraction. IEEE Transaction on Bio-Medical Engineering. 2013;**60**(6)

[13] Mohan J, Krishnaveni V, Guo Y. A new neutrosophic approach of Wiener filtering for MRI denoising. Measurement Science Review. 2013;**13**(4)

[14] Luo S. Filtering medical image using adaptive filter. Engineering in Medicine and Biology Society, 2001. Proceedings of the 23rd Annual International Conference of the IEEE. Vol. 3; 2001. pp. 2727-2729

[15] L Lin, X Meng, X Liang. Reduction of impulse noise in MRI images using block-based adaptive median filter. Medical Imaging Physics and Engineering (ICMIPE), 2013 IEEE International Conference on 19-20 Oct. 2013. 2013. pp.132-134

[16] Hancer E, Ozturk C, Karaboga D. Extraction of brain tumors from MRI images with artificial bee colony based segmentation methodology. 8th International Conference on Electrical Engineering. 2013:516-520

[17] Sivasundari MKS, Siva Kumar R. Performance analysis of image filtering algorithms for MRI images. International Journal of Research in Engineering and Technology. 2014;**3**(5):438-440

[18] Loizou CP, Pantziaris M, Pattichis CS, Seimenis I. Brain MR image normalization in texture analysis of multiple sclerosis. Journal of Biomedical Graphics and Computing. 2012;**3**(1):20-34

[19] Lijun B, Liu W, Zhu Y, Pu Z, Magnin IE. Sparse representation based MRI de-noising with total variation. Signal Processing, 2008. ICSP 2008. 9th International Conference on Oct. 2008; 2008. pp. 2154-2157

[20] Priyadharsini B. A Novel Noise Filtering Technique for De-noising MRI Images. Proceedings of International Conference On Global Innovations In Computing Technology (ICGICT'14), Vol. 2, Special Issue 1, March 2014

[21] Patel K, Mewada H. A review on different image de-noising methods. International Journal on Recent and Innovation Trends in Computing and Communication. 2014;**2**(1): 155-159

[22] Akar S. Determination of optimal parameters for bilateral filter in brain MR image de-noising. Elsevier Applied Soft Computing. 2016;**43**:87-96

Chapter 8

Fourier Velocity Encoded MRI: Acceleration and Velocity Map Estimation

Vinicius C. Rispoli, Joao L.A. Carvalho,
Cristiano J. Miosso and Fabiano A. Soares

Additional information is available at the end of the chapter

http://dx.doi.org/10.5772/intechopen.72531

Abstract

Fourier velocity encoding (FVE) is an alternative to phase contrast imaging (PC). FVE provides considerably higher SNR than PC, due to its higher dimensionality and larger voxel sizes. Furthermore, FVE is robust to partial voluming, as it resolves the velocity distribution within each voxel. FVE data are usually acquired with low spatial resolution, due to scan-time restrictions associated with its higher dimensionality. FVE is capable of providing the velocity distribution associated with a large voxel, but does not directly provides a velocity map. Knowing the velocity distribution on a voxel is important for accurate diagnosis of stenosis in vessels on the scale of spatial resolution. Velocity maps, however, are useful for visualizing the actual blood flow through a vessel and can be used in different studies and diagnosis. In this context, this chapter deals with two aspects of the FVE MRI technique: acceleration and estimation of velocity map. First, are introduced six different acceleration techniques that can be applied to FVE acquisition. Methods such as variable-density sampling and compressive sampling. Then, is proposed a novel method to estimate velocity maps with high spatial resolution from low-resolution FVE data. Finally, it can be concluded that FVE datasets can be acquired in time scale comparable to PC, it contains more velocity information, since it resolves a velocity distribution within a voxel, and also provides an accurate estimation of the velocity map.

Keywords: Fourier velocity encoding, compressive sensing, variable-density sampling, parallel imaging, velocity map estimation

1. Introduction

Cardiovascular diseases are among the main causes of death in both men and women in the United States. Some of these diseases are caused or can be diagnosed by abnormal blood flow in a particular part of the cardiovascular system. For example, atherosclerosis consists of the narrowing of a blood vessel due to the gradual accumulation of lipids, inflammatory cells and connective tissue in the vessel wall [1]. This narrowing alters the local blood flow and may cause flow jets and/or turbulent flow. In these flow jets occur peaks of velocity that are significantly higher than those exhibited at a normal flow. Thus, knowledge of blood flow patterns in the human body is an important component in the research and diagnosis of certain cardiovascular diseases. Currently, two distinct approaches to the study and quantification of blood flow in the human body are available to researchers and clinicians: *in-vivo* direct measurements of the velocity field using velocity-encoded magnetic resonance imaging (MRI) or Doppler ultrasound.

Doppler ultrasound is the gold standard for quantifying blood flow patterns in the clinical environment. The equipment is relatively small, cheap and portable, and is capable of producing measurements in real time with excellent temporal resolution. On the other hand, evaluation by ultrasound is inadequate when there is fat, air, bone, or surgical scar in the acoustic path. Moreover the equipment is strongly user-dependent, since flow measurements are inaccurate when the ultrasound beam cannot be properly aligned with the axis of flow [2, 3].

MRI is capable of three-dimensional visualization of all aspects of a cardiac examination, such as the anatomy of the heart, features in the blood vessels, and also the quantification of velocity in any given vessel. Compared to ultrasound, magnetic resonance imaging does not have the same operator dependence, being able to accurately quantify the correct direction of flow, and does not have the same acoustic limitations related to bones, fat, air or surgical scars.

The current gold standard for MRI flow quantification is phase contrast (PC) [4]. In this technique, a bipolar gradient is aligned to the flow axis to obtain a velocity measurement (approximately the mean [5]) for each voxel of the image. Despite its unrestricted use, phase contrast has some limitations. Phase contrast technique suffers from partial-volume effects when a wide distribution of velocities is contained within a single voxel [6]. This is particularly problematic when flow is turbulent and/or complex (e.g., flow jets due to stenosis) or at the interface between blood and vessel wall (viscous sublayer). This issue is typically addressed by increasing the spatial resolution, which dramatically affects the signal-to-noise ratio (SNR) and increases the scan time. Therefore, PC may be inadequate for estimating the peak velocity of stenotic flow jets and for assessing wall shear rate.

Fourier velocity encoded (FVE) MRI [7] is a magnetic resonance velocity quantification technique which is as an alternative to phase contrast imaging, since real-time FVE is the MRI equivalent to spectral-Doppler ultrasound [8]. In this technique, the acquired measurements have a considerably higher signal-to-noise ratio than those acquired with phase contrast, due to its high-dimensional data set and also to its larger voxels. In addition, different from PC data, FVE does not suffer from partial volume effects, since for each voxel a velocity distribution is measured. So this technique can accurately diagnose vessels stenosis on low spatial resolution. The data set measured with this technique is usually obtained with very low spatial resolution. This is due to restrictions associated with its high dimensionality, which can lead to long acquisitions time. Thus, FVE is not a popular technique in the clinical environment that requires exams to be performed as fast as possible. On the other hand, it has been shown that the FVE acquisition can be accelerated. For example, FVE acquisition using rapid spiral sampling in *k*-space is a fast and reliable alternative to accurately measure velocity peaks in blood flow jets or to obtain hemodynamic parameters [9].

In this context, this chapter deals with two aspects of the FVE MRI technique: acceleration and estimation of velocity map. First, are introduced six different important acceleration techniques that can be applied to FVE acquisition and are related to the use of variable-density sampling, which may be used along spatial k-space and velocity k-space, partial Fourier acquisition along velocity k-space, temporal acceleration methods such as UNFOLD and k-t BLAST, parallel imaging methods and compressive sampling.

Finally, since FVE does not provide the actual velocity map associated with the flow, is proposed a novel method to velocity maps estimation with high spatial resolution from low-resolution FVE data. The proposed method is based on the mathematical model of the FVE distribution, $s(x, y, v)$, and involves solving a PDE-constrained optimization related to the Navier-Stokes equation.

2. Magnetic resonance flow imaging

MRI is a modality uniquely capable of imaging all aspects of cardiovascular disease, and is a potential "one-stop shop" for cardiovascular health assessment. MRI can generate cross-sectional images in any plane (including oblique planes), and can also measure blood flow. The image acquisition is based on using strong magnetic fields and non-ionizing radiation in the radio frequency range, which are harmless to the patient. MR is used to image hydrogen nuclei, because of its abundance in the human body. Spinning charged particles (or "spins"), such as hydrogen nuclei, act like a tiny bar magnet, presenting a very small magnetic field, emanating from the south pole to the north pole. In this section we introduce the mathematical formalism of MR imaging and flow imaging.

2.1. Mathematical formalism

The acquired MR signal $s(t)$ at a particular time instant corresponds to a sample of the Fourier transform $M(k_x, k_y)$ of the excited magnetization $m(x, y)$:

$$M(k_x, k_y) = \int_x \int_y m(x, y) e^{-j2\pi(k_x x + k_y y)}\, dx\, dy. \tag{1}$$

The Fourier coordinates k_x and k_y vary with time, according to the zeroth moment of the readout gradients G_x and G_y:

$$k_x(t) = \frac{\gamma}{2\pi} \int_0^t G_x(\tau)\, d\tau \tag{2}$$

$$k_y(t) = \frac{\gamma}{2\pi} \int_0^t G_y(\tau)\, d\tau. \tag{3}$$

This formalism can be generalized for any combination of G_x, G_y, and G_z gradients:

$$M\left(\vec{k}_r\right) = \int_{\vec{r}} m\left(\vec{r}\right) \cdot e^{-j2\pi \vec{k}_r \cdot \vec{r}}\, d\vec{r} \tag{4}$$

$$\vec{k}_r(t) = \frac{\gamma}{2\pi} \int_0^t \vec{G}_r(\tau)\, d\tau, \tag{5}$$

where $\vec{G}_r$ is the oblique gradient resulting from the combination of the G_x, G_y and G_z gradients, and $\vec{r}$ is its corresponding axis along which the linear variation in magnetic field intensity is realized.

Given a spatial position function $\vec{r}(t)$ and a magnetic field gradient $\vec{G}_r(t)$, the magnetization phase is:

$$\phi\left(\vec{r}, t\right) = \gamma \int_0^t \vec{G}_r(\tau) \cdot \vec{r}\,(\tau)\, d\tau, \tag{6}$$

For static spins, $\vec{r}\,(t)$ is constant ($\vec{r}$), and this becomes:

$$\phi = \gamma\, \vec{r} \cdot \int_0^t \vec{G}_r(\tau)\, d\tau \tag{7}$$

$$= 2\pi\, \vec{k}_r \cdot \vec{r}\,, \tag{8}$$

as in the exponential in Eq. (4).

2.2. Principles of MR flow imaging

The basic principles of quantitative flow measurement using magnetic resonance were first proposed by Singer [10] and Hahn [11] in the late 1950s. However, clinical applications of MR flow quantification were not reported until the early 1980s [12–15]. Current MR flow imaging methods are based on the fact that spins moving at a constant velocity accrue a phase proportional to the velocity times the first moment of the gradient waveform along the direction in which they are moving.

For spins moving along the $\vec{r}$-axis with a constant velocity $\vec{v}$, and initial position $\vec{r}_0$, we can write $\vec{r}\,(t) = \vec{r}_0 + \vec{v}t$. Rewriting Eq. (6), for $t = t_0$:

$$\phi = \gamma \int_0^{t_0} \vec{G}_r(t) \cdot \left(\vec{r}_0 + \vec{v}t\right) dt \tag{9}$$

$$= \gamma \vec{r}_0 \cdot \int_0^{t_0} \vec{G}_r(t)\, dt + \gamma \vec{v} \cdot \int_0^{t_0} \vec{G}_r(t)\, t\, dt \tag{10}$$

$$= \gamma \vec{r}_0 \cdot \vec{M}_0 + \gamma \vec{v} \cdot \vec{M}_1, \tag{11}$$

http://dx.doi.org/10.5772/intechopen.72531

where $\vec{M}_0$ and $\vec{M}_1$ are the zeroth and first moments of the $\vec{r}$-gradient waveform at the time of signal acquisitions ("echo time", or "time to echo" (TE)), respectively. Thus, if a gradient with null zeroth moment is used (e.g., a bipolar gradient, aligned with $\vec{v}$), the phase accrued for a constant velocity spin is $\phi = \gamma \vec{v} \cdot \vec{M}_1$.

Therefore, if a bipolar gradient waveform is played between the excitation and the readout, the phase measured in a pixel of the acquired image is directly proportional to the velocity of the spins contained within its corresponding voxel. However, factors other than flow (such as inhomogeneities of the magnetic field) may cause additional phase shifts that would cause erroneous interpretation of the local velocity [16].

2.2.1. *Phase contrast*

The phase contrast method addresses the problem mentioned above by using two gradient-echo data acquisitions in which the first moment of the bipolar gradient waveform is varied between measurements [4]. So from Eq. (11) it is possible to obtain time-dependent velocity measures in all three spatial directions. Then for a fixed time and direction, e.g. velocity in z-axis, the through-plane velocity in each voxel is measured as:

$$v_z(x,y) = \frac{\phi_a(x,y) - \phi_b(x,y)}{\gamma(M_1^a - M_1^b)}, \tag{12}$$

where $\phi_a(x,y)$ and $\phi_b(x,y)$ are the phase images acquired in each acquisition, and M_1^a and M_1^b are the first moment of the bipolar gradients used in each acquisition.

2.2.2. *Fourier velocity encoding*

While phase contrast provides a single velocity measurement associated with each voxel, Fourier velocity encoding [7] provides a velocity histogram for each spatial location, which is a measurement of the velocity distribution within each voxel.

FVE involves phase-encoding along a velocity dimension. Instead of only two acquisitions, as in phase contrast, multiple acquisitions are performed, and a bipolar gradient with a different amplitude (and first moment) is used in each acquisition. Eq. (11) can be rewritten as:

$$\phi\left(\vec{r}, \vec{v}, t\right) = 2\pi\left(\vec{k}_r \cdot \vec{r} + \vec{k}_v \cdot \vec{v}\right), \tag{13}$$

where $\vec{k}_v$ is the velocity frequency variable associated with $\vec{v}$, and is proportional to the first moment of $\vec{G}_r(t)$:

$$\vec{k}_v = \frac{\gamma}{2\pi} \vec{M}_1. \tag{14}$$

Each voxel of the two-dimensional image is associated with a distribution of velocities. This three-dimensional function $m(x,y,v)$ is associated with a three-dimensional Fourier space

$M(k_x, k_y, k_v)$. Thus, an extra dimension is added to k-space, and multiple acquisitions are required to cover the entire k_x-k_y-k_v space (**Figure 1**). In order to move along k_v, a bipolar gradient with the appropriate amplitude (and first moment) is played before the k_x-k_y readout gradients, in each acquisition. Placing the bipolar gradient along the z-axis will encode through-plane velocities. Placing the bipolar gradient along x or y will encode in-plane velocities. Oblique flow can be encoded using a combination of bipolar gradients along the x, y and z axes.

Each acquisition along k_v is called a velocity encode. The number of required velocity encodes depends on the desired velocity resolution and velocity field-of-view (the maximum range of velocities measured without aliasing). For example, to obtain a 25 cm/s resolution over a 600 cm/s field-of-view, 24 velocity encodes are needed. The spatial-velocity distribution, $m(x, y, v)$, is obtained by inverse Fourier transforming the acquired data, $M(k_x, k_y, k_v)$. If cine imaging [17] is used, measurements are also time resolved, resulting in a four-dimensional dataset: $m(x, y, v, t)$.

2.3. FVE signal model

2DFT phase contrast provides two 2-dimensional functions, $m(x, y)$ and $v_z(x, y)$, the magnitude and velocity maps, respectively. For simplicity we are assuming that the through-plane velocity map is in the z direction. If these maps are measured with sufficiently high spatial resolution, and flow is laminar, one can assume that each voxel contains only one velocity, and therefore the spatial-velocity distribution associated with the object is approximately:

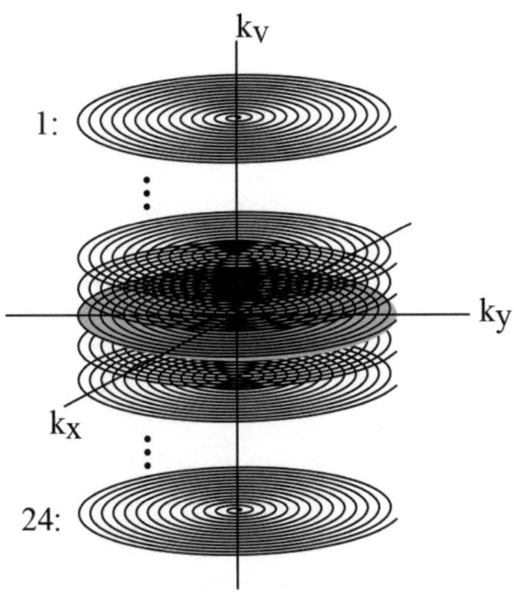

Figure 1. Spiral FVE k-space sampling scheme. The dataset corresponding to each temporal frame is a stack-of-spirals in k_x-k_y-k_v space. Each spiral acquisition corresponds to a different k_v encode level.

$$s(x,y,v) = m(x,y) \times \delta(\ v - v_z(x,y)\ ), \tag{15}$$

where $\delta(v)$ is the Dirac delta function.

In 2DFT FVE, k-space data is truncated to a rectangular cuboid in k_x-k_y-k_v space. The associated object domain spatial-velocity blurring can be modeled as a convolution of the true object distribution, $s(x,y,v)$, with $\mathrm{sinc}(x/\Delta x)$, $\mathrm{sinc}(y/\Delta y)$, and $\mathrm{sinc}(v/\Delta v)$, where Δx and Δy are the spatial resolutions along the x and y axes, respectively, and Δv is the velocity resolution, as follows:

$$\widehat{s}(x,y,v) = [m(x,y) \times \delta(\ v - v_z(x,y)\ )]*\mathrm{sinc}\left(\frac{x}{\Delta x}\right)*\mathrm{sinc}\left(\frac{y}{\Delta y}\right)*\mathrm{sinc}\left(\frac{v}{\Delta v}\right), \tag{16}$$

where $\widehat{s}(x,y,v)$ is the measured object distribution and $*$ denotes convolution. This is equivalent to:

$$\widehat{s}(x,y,v) = \left[m(x,y) \times \mathrm{sinc}\left(\frac{v - v_z(x,y)}{\Delta v}\right)\right] * \left[\mathrm{sinc}\left(\frac{x}{\Delta x}\right) \times \mathrm{sinc}\left(\frac{y}{\Delta y}\right)\right]. \tag{17}$$

On the other hand, spiral FVE acquisitions follows a stack-of-spirals pattern in k_x-k_y-k_v space (**Figure 1**), then k-space data is truncated to a cylinder, i.e., a circle along k_x-k_y (with diameter $1/\Delta r$), and a rect function along k_v (with width $1/\Delta v$), where Δr and Δv are the prescribed spatial and velocity resolutions, respectively. Using the same approach we used for 2DFT FVE, the associated object domain spatial-velocity blurring in spiral FVE can be modeled as a convolution of the true object distribution, $s(x,y,v)$, with $\mathrm{jinc}\left(\sqrt{x^2+y^2}/\Delta r\right)$ and $\mathrm{sinc}(v/\Delta v)$, resulting in:

$$\begin{aligned}\widehat{s}\,(x,y,v) &= [m(x,y) \times \delta(\ v - v_z(x,y)\ )]*\mathrm{sinc}\left(\frac{v}{\Delta v}\right)*\mathrm{jinc}\left(\frac{\sqrt{x^2+y^2}}{\Delta r}\right)\\ &= \left[m(x,y) \times \mathrm{sinc}\left(\frac{v - v_z(x,y)}{\Delta v}\right)\right]*\mathrm{jinc}\left(\frac{\sqrt{x^2+y^2}}{\Delta r}\right),\end{aligned} \tag{18}$$

where $\mathrm{jinc}(z) = J_1(\pi z)/(2z)$ and $J_1(z)$ is the Bessel function of the first kind and first order. These approaches for deriving FVE data from high-resolution velocity maps will be used for the map estimation purposes.

3. Acceleration of FVE

FVE datasets are multidimensional, which makes this method particularly suitable for accelerated acquisition. Variable-density sampling may be used along spatial k-space, and also along velocity k-space. Partial Fourier acquisition along velocity k-space can be used to reduce scan time by nearly 50%. Temporal acceleration methods such as UNFOLD and k-t BLAST have been demonstrated with FVE. Parallel imaging methods have also been shown to work well with FVE. Also FVE is optimally suited for acquisition acceleration using compressed sensing. This section introduces each of these acceleration methods.

3.1. Variable-density sampling of spatial k-space

Magnetic resonance imaging can be accelerated using variable-density sampling of k-space. This is typically implemented by using a sampling pattern that satisfies the Nyquist criterion at the low spatial frequencies, and undersamples the high spatial frequencies. In other words, the effective field-of-view (FOV) is varied from the desired FOV at the center of k-space to a reduced FOV at the periphery [18]. The general hypothesis is that artifacts from undersampling the periphery of k-space will be negligible, because the energy of high frequency components is typically much lower than that of low frequency components. Variable-density spirals can increase spatiotemporal resolution and improve accuracy in flow quantitation [19]. The spatial aliasing resulting from variable-density spiral sampling is incoherent, and, in the regions-of-interest (e.g., cardiac chambers, valves, great vessels), it typically originates from static or slow moving material located at the periphery of the spatial FOV (e.g., chest wall). FVE resolves the distribution of velocities within the voxel, thus moderate low-velocity aliasing artifacts generally do not affect one's ability to calculate diagnostically important parameters—such as peak velocity and acceleration—from the time-velocity distribution.

The use of variable-density spirals for acceleration of slice-selective FVE with spiral readouts is illustrated in **Figure 2**. A single-shot uniform-density spiral readout was replaced with a multi-shot variable-density spiral acquisition. The use of multi-shot acquisitions provides the possibility of multi-dimensional temporal acceleration, and allows reduction of readout duration and TR, which reduce off-resonance artifacts and temporal aliasing, respectively. The use of a shorter TR also allows improving the temporal resolution. The data in **Figure 2a** was obtained using a single-interleave 8 ms readout uniform-density spiral design [20, 21]. The variable-density design used three 4 ms spiral interleaves, and provided higher spatial resolution and reduced off-resonance artifacts, and thus better spatial localization of flow (**Figure 2b**) [9]. Some aliasing artifacts were observed in spatial domain (see asterisk), but these were not observed in the time-velocity distributions. A fully sampled reference is shown in **Figure 2c**, for comparison.

3.2. Variable-density sampling of velocity k-space

Variable-density sampling of velocity k-space was first demonstrated by DiCarlo et al. [22] using real-time FVE. Real-time FVE (also known as MR Doppler or one-shot FVE) [8, 23–25] utilizes cylindrical excitation to restrict the spatial field-of-view to a one-dimensional beam. An oscillating readout gradient simultaneously encodes spatial position and velocity along the axis of the beam. Variable-density sampling of velocity k-space has also been demonstrated using slice-selective FVE [26]. Variable-density sampling along the velocity dimension may be used to improve the velocity resolution and/or increase the velocity field-of-view. However, conventional non-Cartesian reconstruction methods such as gridding and direct Fourier

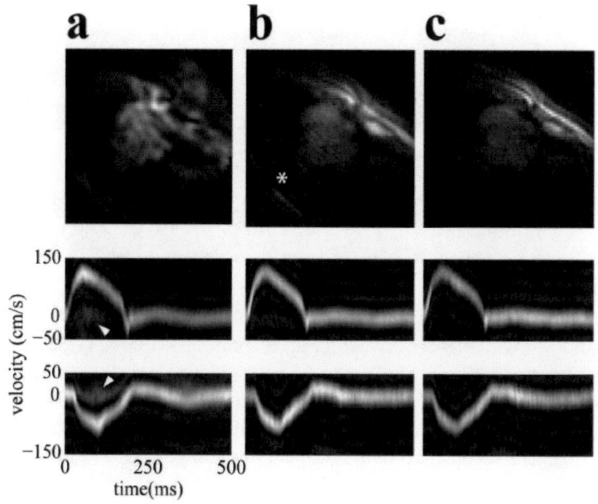

Figure 2. Effect of variable-density sampling of spatial k-space on image quality and spatial localization of flow: (a) uniform-density design; (b) variable-density design; (c) ground truth reference. Top row: spatial images from the first cardiac phase; center row: time-velocity distributions measured at the aortic valve; bottom row: time-velocity distributions measured in the descending aorta. The use of higher spatial resolution and shorter readout duration improves the spatial localization of flow, which is identified by the reduced signal from static material in the time-velocity histograms (see arrows). Some aliasing artifacts were observed in spatial domain (see asterisk), but these were not observed in the time-velocity distributions.

transform (DrFT) do not adequately deal with the associated undersampling artifacts. Alternatively, reconstruction of variable-density FVE may be performed using variable-width sinc interpolation with dynamic field-of-view centering [26]. **Figure 3** illustrates the use of variable-density sampling along velocity k-space for accelerating slice-selective FVE [26]. The reconstruction scheme using variable-width sinc interpolation with dynamic field-of-view centering exhibits negligible aliasing artifacts compared to conventional gridding (see arrows). There is also no noticeable loss of velocity resolution compared with the small velocity FOV ground truth reference. Note the improvement in velocity resolution compared with the large FOV uniform-density result.

3.3. Partial Fourier acquisition of velocity k-space

Partial Fourier acquisition and reconstruction exploits the conjugate symmetry property of the Fourier transform of real-valued signals. The method involves acquiring slightly greater than one half of k-space, and synthesizing the missing data using a combination of conjugate synthesis and background phase correction. A narrow strip of k-space is acquired with symmetric coverage in order to estimate this smoothly-varying background phase. The fastest and most widely used method of partial Fourier reconstruction is homodyne detection [27]. Acquisition time in FVE can be reduced by 30–40% using partial Fourier acceleration along the velocity dimension. This consists in acquiring only slightly more than half of the k_v encodings, and synthesizing the missing data using homodyne reconstruction. This has been successfully used in FVE for scan time reduction, without significant loss of velocity resolution. This

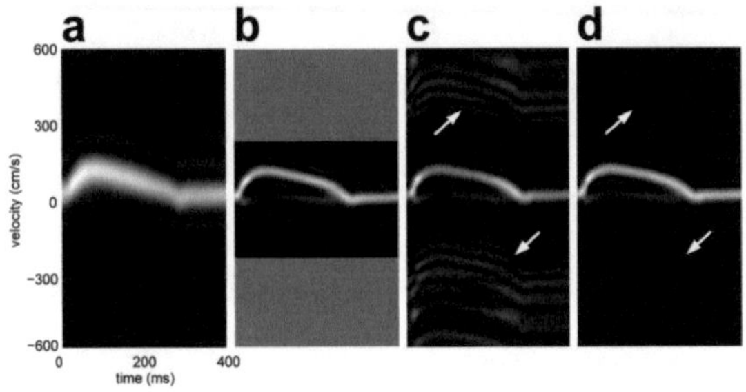

Figure 3. *In vivo* demonstration of variable-density sampling of velocity k-space. Velocity distributions were measured using slice-selective spiral FVE at the aortic valve plane of a healthy volunteer using: (a) uniform-density sampling, large FOV; (b) uniform-density sampling, small FOV (ground truth); (c) variable-density sampling, reconstructed using conventional gridding; and (d) variable-density sampling, reconstructed using variable-width sinc interpolation with dynamic field-of-view centering. The reconstruction scheme using variable-width sinc interpolation with dynamic field-of-view centering reduces undersampling artifacts (arrows), and shows velocity resolution equivalent to that of the ground truth reference.

approach has been demonstrated in studies with healthy volunteers [8, 20, 21] and patients [20, 21, 25, 28], and in phantom experiments [22]. The feasibility of reducing scan time in FVE using partial Fourier acquisition is illustrated in **Figure 4**. Up to 42% of the acquired data (along velocity k-space) was discarded and then synthesized using homodyne reconstruction. The results show 71 and 60% improvement in velocity resolution using this approach, when imaging the aortic valves of a healthy volunteer and of a patient with aortic stenosis. Partial Fourier performs well in both healthy volunteer and patient studies, and no significant loss of resolution or artifacts is noticed [20, 21].

3.4. Temporal acceleration

In dynamic MRI, view sharing [29] is commonly used to increase the number of temporal frames. Artifacts and loss of temporal resolution due to view sharing can be avoided or corrected using temporal acceleration techniques, such as UNFOLD [30, 31] and k-t BLAST [32]. UNFOLD reduces scan time by making efficient use of k-t space, and can be very successful in the context of slice-selective FVE due to the high dimensionality of this imaging method. The use of UNFOLD for acceleration of FVE was first demonstrated by Macgowan and Madore [33], and further investigated by Carvalho and Nayak [9, 20, 21]. **Figure 5** illustrates an implementation of the UNFOLD method specially designed for slice-selective FVE with spiral readouts [9, 20, 21]. A view-ordering scheme that reduces overlap in v-f space was designed (v denotes the through-plane velocity dimension, and f denotes temporal frequency). **Figure 2a** shows the undersampled data in both *v–f* and *v–t* domains (where t denotes time). The aliasing signal is filtered using a two-dimensional filter (**Figure 5a**). This filter has a bandwidth of 107 Hz for velocities below ±150 cm/s. For higher velocities, the bandwidth varies from 69 to 30 Hz. This results in effective temporal resolutions of 9.3 and 14.5–33.3 ms, respectively. The temporal resolution is lower for higher velocities, but this may prove unnoticeable, as the velocity distribution of high-velocity flow jets within large voxels is typically temporally smooth. For comparison, the temporal resolution with view sharing

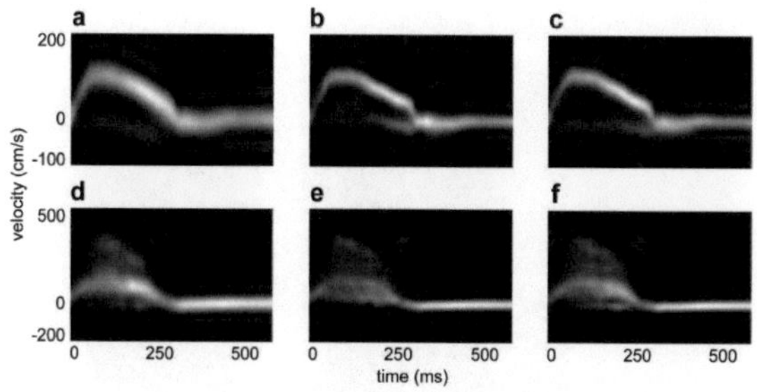

Figure 4. Evaluation of partial k-space reconstruction along the velocity dimension, in aortic valve studies of a healthy volunteer (a–c) and a patient with aortic stenosis (d–f). Homodyne reconstruction performs well in both healthy volunteer (b) and patient (e) studies, improving the velocity resolution by 71 and 60%, respectively. Full k-space distributions with the same number of velocity-encode samples are shown for comparison (a,d), as well as the fully sampled datasets (c,f).

would be 50 ms for all velocities (**Figure 5d**). The remaining narrow-bandwidth aliasing components at ±20 and ±40 Hz are filtered using a tight zero-phase one-dimensional notch filter along the temporal dimension (**Figure 5b**). The final results show that this temporal acceleration scheme is capable of achieving 6-fold acceleration in multi-interleaf spiral FVE, without noticeable loss of temporal resolution, and without introducing significant artifacts (**Figure 5c**). View-sharing (**Figure 5d**), on the other hand, is equivalent to a moving-average low-pass filter, which reduces the temporal frequency bandwidth (dashed arrows), and causes loss of temporal resolution, perceived as blurring along time (circled).

3.5. Parallel imaging

Spatial aliasing due to undersampling of slice-selective FVE can be reduced using parallel imaging methods such as SENSE [34] and SPIRiT [35]. Parallel imaging is an acceleration approach that uses data from multiple coils to reduce aliasing artifacts due to undersampling of spatial k-space [34]. Steeden et al. was able to accelerate slice-selective spiral FVE by a factor of four using SENSE [28]. Lyra-Leite et al. used two-dimensional and three-dimensional SPIRiT to accelerate slice-selective spiral FVE by factors of two and four, respectively [36, 37]. In the velocity distributions measured using slice-selective FVE, aliasing due to spatial undersampling typically results in increased signal at $v = 0$ cm/s, since the majority of the aliasing signal is associated with static material. **Figure 6** illustrates the use of two-dimensional SPIRiT to accelerate slice-selective spiral FVE by a factor of two [36]. SPIRiT is able to considerably reduce aliasing artifacts, while not introducing significant artifacts (see error images).

3.6. Compressive sensing

Compressive sensing (CS) has been used in MRI [38] context for a while in different applications, such as fMRI images [39], PC-MRI velocity maps [40] and also FVE distributions [41, 42]. Basically, is a set of theories and methods that establish the conditions under which a signal can be reconstructed based on a limited number of linear measurements. It also states different procedures for signal reconstruction, provided that these conditions are properly met [43–46]. For a successful image reconstruction using CS the desired image must satisfy three

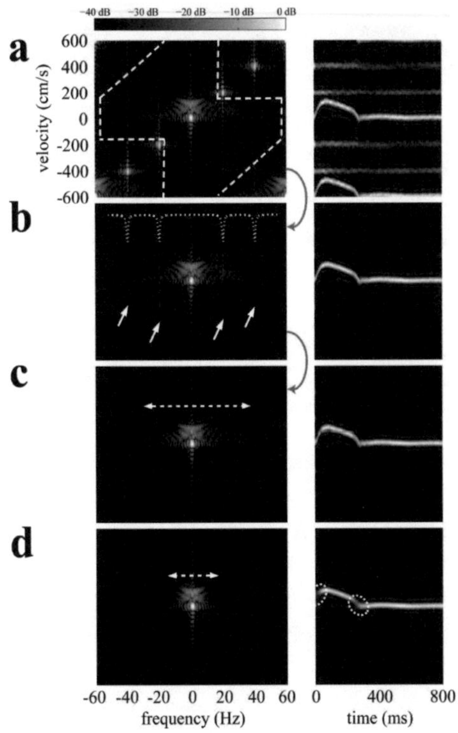

Figure 5. Temporal acceleration compared with view sharing in (left) v-f space and (right) v-t space: (a) undersampled data; (b) with two-dimensional filtering; (c) with two-dimensional and notch filtering; and (d) with view sharing. The two-dimensional filter (dashed lines) removes a majority of the aliasing, and the notch filter (dotted line) removes the remaining aliasing signal (solid arrows). This approach removes aliasing components without noticeable loss of temporal resolution. View sharing reduces the temporal frequency bandwidth (dashed arrows) and causes temporal blurring (circles).

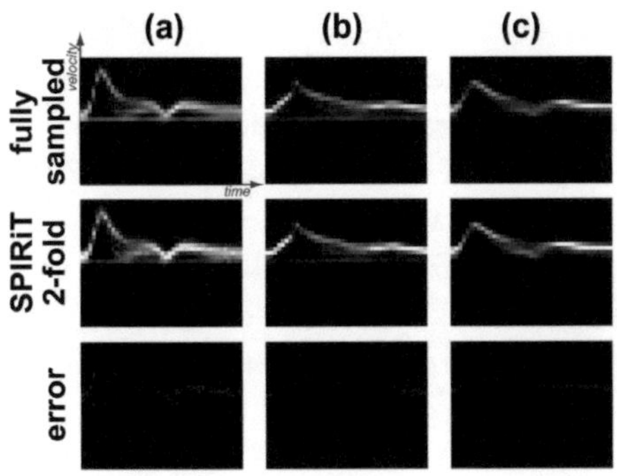

Figure 6. Time-velocity distributions from select voxels, reconstructed using twofold accelerated two-dimensional SPIRiT (center row), in comparison with the fully sampled reference (top row): (a) right external carotid artery; (b) right internal carotid artery; and (c) left carotid bifurcation.

conditions: (1) must have a sparse representation in a known transform domain, (2) artifacts caused by k-space undersampling must be incoherent in the sparsifying transform domain and (3) must be reconstructed by a nonlinear method that enforces both sparsity of the image representation and consistency of the reconstruction with the acquired samples [38].

http://dx.doi.org/10.5772/intechopen.72531

FVE data is suitable for CS application, since the information contained in images with different velocity encodes is highly redundant differing only where flow occurs. Therefore, through spatial finite differencing operations FVE dataset have a sparse representation [38, 42].

The original CS reconstruction problem is a NP-hard problem, generally of combinatorial complexity [46–48], and is not viable except for very low-dimensional cases. Thus, the original problem can be relaxed and a precise reconstruction can be achieved using the following non-linear constrained optimization problem:

$$\mathbf{f}^* = \text{argmin}_{\mathbf{f}} \|\mathbf{Tf}\|_{\ell_p}^p \text{ s. t. } \mathbf{Mf} = \mathbf{s}, \tag{19}$$

where $0 < p \leq 1$, $\mathbf{T}$ is the sparsifying transform, $\mathbf{M}$ is the acquisition process matrix, $\mathbf{f}$ is the desired image, $\mathbf{s}$ is the acquired signal and

$$\|\mathbf{f}\|_{\ell_p} = \left(\sum_{n=1}^{N} |f_n|^p \right)^{1/p}. \tag{20}$$

Usually in most CS applications the value of p is set to $p = 1$, but it has been shown that for ℓ_p-minimization (with $0 < p < 1$) requires fewer measurements than ℓ_1 [46]. In order to reconstruct MR data based on ℓ_p-minimization, one can use the algorithm described by Miosso et al. [45].

Other possible ways to enhance signal reconstruction in CS, both in terms of reducing the number of required measurements and in terms of improving image quality for a fixed number of measurements, include the use of support prior information extracted from structural knowledge, previous frames or previous slices [39, 46], and the use of information extracted using machine learning techniques [49, 50]. Other alternative optimization problems are also desired in the context of noisy measurements, in which case, for example, the equality constraint in Problem 19 is replaced by an inequality such as $\|\mathbf{Mf} - \mathbf{s}\|_{\ell_2} \leq \varepsilon$, with ε being a tolerance to noise [47, 48] — the higher the value of ε, the higher the number of measurements required for reconstruction.

In this context, has been shown by Marinelli et al. [51] and Hilbert et al. [42] that CS can also be used as an acceleration technique for FVE datasets and the acquisition can be made in time scale comparable to the gold standard phase contrast. So it is possible to obtain meaningful velocity spectra in small vessels in clinical time while regular phase contrast can provide only mean velocity maps [42].

4. Estimating velocity maps from FVE distributions

In this section will be discussed a methodology to estimate the velocity map based on the FVE velocity distribution. It has been shown in Section 2.3 that FVE velocity distribution signal model $\hat{s}(x, y, v)$ is related to the actual velocity map $v_z(x, y)$ through the relation

$$\hat{s}(x, y, v) = \left[m(x, y) \times \text{sinc}\left(\frac{v - v_z(x, y)}{\Delta v} \right) \right] * \Psi(x, y), \tag{21}$$

where $\Psi(x, y)$ is a point spread function associated with k-space truncation data. This provide a first relation between the FVE measured velocity distribution and the velocity map. On the other hand, blood can be ideally modeled as an incompressible Newtonian fluid. Then, blood flow can be predicted using the Navier-Stokes equation

$$\rho\left(\frac{\partial \mathbf{v}}{\partial t} + \mathbf{v}\cdot\nabla\mathbf{v}\right) = -\nabla p + \mu\nabla^2\mathbf{v}, \tag{22}$$

where $\mathbf{v} = \left(v_x, v_y, v_z\right)$ is the velocity vector, ρ is the blood density, μ is the whole blood viscosity and ∇^2 is the Laplacian differential operator. Then, ideally the desired velocity map must satisfy the flow physics model. Therefore, for a fixed instant of time, a velocity map can be estimated from a measured FVE dataset $f(x, y, v)$, with K velocity encodes, through the following PDE-constrained optimization problem

$$\min_{v_z}\sum_{k=1}^{K}\int_\Omega\left\{f(\mathbf{x}, v_k) - \left[m(\mathbf{x})\times \mathrm{sinc}\left(\frac{v_k - v_z}{\Delta v}\right)\right]*\Psi(\mathbf{x})\right\}^2 dA\ \mathrm{s.t.}\rho\mathbf{v}\cdot\nabla\mathbf{v} = -\nabla p + \mu\nabla^2\mathbf{v}, \tag{23}$$

where $\mathbf{x} = (x, y)$ is the position vector and v_k is a velocity encode.

In order to solve Eq. (23) the Navier-Stokes equation must be discretized. Since the interest here is in a proof-of-concept velocity map estimation based on only one component of the velocity vector, a bidimensional version of the physics model solver was used. Fluid is assumed incompressible, so the steady 2D Navier-Stokes-continuity dimensionless system of equations [52],

$$\mathbf{v}\cdot\nabla\mathbf{v} = -\nabla p + \frac{1}{\mathrm{Re}}\nabla^2\mathbf{v} \text{ and } \nabla\cdot\mathbf{v} = 0, \tag{24}$$

was discretized using the Finite Element Method [53], where Re is the Reynolds number [52], $\mathbf{v} = v_x\mathbf{i} + v_z\mathbf{j} \in \mathrm{IR}^2$ is the velocity field and p is the pressure. Discretization is made using residues functions based on the governing equations' weak form Gresho and Sani [53]

$$R_c(\mathbf{v}) = \int_\Omega(\nabla\cdot\mathbf{v})\phi d\Omega \tag{25}$$

and

$$R_m(\mathbf{v}, p) = \int_\Omega(\mathbf{v}\cdot\nabla\mathbf{v})\cdot\Psi d\Omega + \int_\Omega \mathrm{s} : \nabla\Psi d\Omega - \int_\Gamma(\mathbf{n}\cdot\mathrm{s})\cdot\Psi d\Gamma, \tag{26}$$

where $\phi \in \mathrm{IR}$, $\Psi \in \mathrm{IR}^2$ are test functions, and $\sigma = -p\mathbf{I} + \mathrm{Re}^{-1}\left[\nabla\mathbf{v} + \nabla\mathbf{v}^T\right]$ the Newtonian stress tensor [52].

Discretizatized equations are written as a linear system $\mathbf{Jc} = \mathbf{r}$, where $\mathbf{J}$ is a matrix given by the residues' Jacobian, $\mathbf{r}$ is a vector given by the residues and $\mathbf{c}$ is the solution vector containing velocity and pressure. Now the minimization problem given by Eq. (23) can be written as

$$\min_{\mathbf{v}_z} \sum_{k=1}^{K} \left\| \mathbf{f}_k - \left[\mathbf{m} \times \text{sinc}\left(\frac{v_k - \mathbf{v}_z}{\Delta v} \right) \right] * \Psi \right\|_{\ell_2}^2 + \lambda \| \mathbf{J}[\mathbf{v}_x; \mathbf{v}_z; \mathbf{p}] - \mathbf{r} \|_{\ell_2}^2, \tag{27}$$

where $\mathbf{c} = [\mathbf{v}_x; \mathbf{v}_z; \mathbf{p}]$ is the solution vector written in a stacked form and $\mathbf{m}$ is a spin density map with high spatial resolution.

In order to validate the proposed constrained optimization (Eq. (27)) an simple experiment was carried out. To do so, a FVE dataset was simulated from an acquired PC dataset, then the optimization was solved and finally the resultant velocity map was compared with the acquired PC velocity map qualitatively and quantitatively.

First, high-spatial-resolution four-dimensional PC data of a pulsatile carotid flow phantom (Phantoms by Design, Inc., Bothell, WA) were obtained using a 3DFT SPGR pulse sequence. The scan parameters were: $0.5 \times 0.5 \times 1$ mm^3 spatial resolution; field-of-view $4.0 \times 3.5 \times 5.0$ cm^3; TR 11.4 ms; flip angle 8.5°; temporal resolution 91.2 ms; VENC 50 cm/s; 40 min per scan; 9 NEX. The data were acquired on a GE Discovery MR750 3T system, with a 32-channel receive-only head coil array (Nova Medical, Inc., Wilmington, MA, USA). The through-slab (z) axis was oriented along the S/I direction. The phantom's pulse cycle was set to 60 bpm. The velocity map for each spatial axis—u_{pc}, v_{pc}, and w_{pc}—was reconstructed using data from all channels of the receive coil array. The lumen was segmented by manually outlining the vessel borders from a stack of 2D axial images, obtained from the reconstructed 3D volume.

Then simulated spiral FVE distributions were derived from the acquired phase contrast data using the signal model presented in Eq. (21). Simulated data was generated only for the through-axis velocity component (v_z), and for a cardiac phase corresponding to the phantom's mid-systole. The 9-NEX PC dataset was used in this process, so that the FVE distributions were computed from low-noise velocity maps (as in Carvalho et al. [54]). This is because FVE has considerably higher SNR than PC in general, due to its higher dimensionality and larger voxel size. Finally, two different spiral FVE distributions were obtained for each slice of the volume with $\Delta r = 2$ mm spatial resolution: one using the proposed method and the other one using the method proposed by Rispoli and Carvalho [55]. The velocity resolution was set to $\Delta v = 10$ cm/s, over a 120 cm/s velocity field-of-view.

About the discretization of the Navier-Stokes equations, lumen manually outlined was used to define computational mesh and simulation grid was designed with 1.0×0.5 mm^2 element resolution using Q_2/P_{-1} elements. Phantom's blood-mimicking fluid (with Reynolds number $Re = 110$) was assumed to be Newtonian and incompressible. PC-MRI velocity profile was set at the inlet together with no-slip boundary condition.

The optimization problem given by Eq. (27) was then solved using a alternating minimization technique [56]. Left side part was solved using a standard non-linear least squares algorithm and the physics model part of the optimization was solved using Newton's method [53].

Figure 7 presents the results of the validation experiment using the phase contrast velocity map acquired at the pulsatile carotid flow phantom's bifurcation. The velocity maps estimated from the simulated low spatial resolution FVE data are very similar (qualitatively) to the reference map. At first glance one can say that the velocity map obtained using the technique proposed by Rispoli and Carvalho [55] (**Figure 7c**) is more similar to the acquired PC-MRI

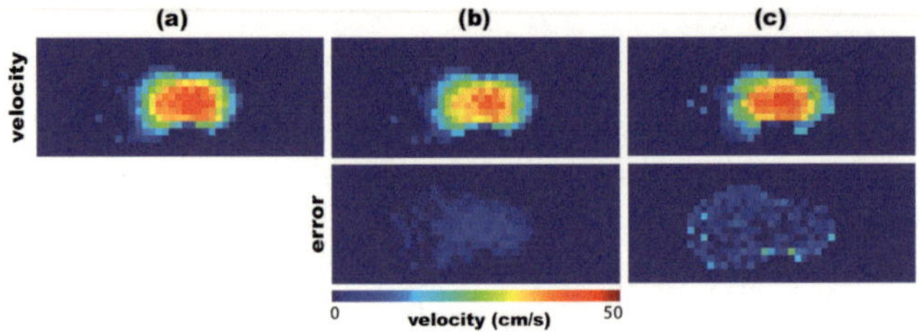

Figure 7. Validation experiment using a pulsatile carotid flow phantom: (a) reference phase contrast velocity map, measured at the phantom's bifurcation; (b) velocity map estimated from the simulated low-resolution spiral FVE data with $\Delta r = 2$ mm spatial resolution with the proposed method (and associated error percentages); and (c) velocity map estimated from the simulated low-resolution spiral FVE data with $\Delta r = 2$ mm spatial resolution with the method proposed by Rispoli and Carvalho [55] (and associated error percentages).

velocity map. However the error images show that the velocity map obtained using the technique proposed in this work (**Figure 7b**) was more accurate than the one obtained with the other method (**Figure 7c**).

Moreover, a quantitative comparison was performed based on the signal-to-error ratio (SER). The acquired phase contrast velocity field, v_{pc}, was used as the ground-truth "signal"; consequently, the estimation error is the difference between the estimated velocity field, v_e, and the ground-truth field, v_{pc}. Thus, the SER is calculated (in decibels) as:

$$\mathrm{SER}_{\vec{v}} = 10 \log_{10}\left(\frac{\sum_{i,j} \left\| v_{\mathrm{pc}}(i,j) \right\|^2}{\sum_{i,j} \left\| v_e(i,j) - v_{\mathrm{pc}}(i,j) \right\|^2}\right), \tag{28}$$

Finally, the proposed method measured SER, relative to the PC reference, was 44.63 dB while the technique proposed in Rispoli and Carvalho [55] achieved 28.68 dB. Showing that the proposed optimization given by Eq. (27) is more consistent with the actual velocity map than the previous method proposed.

These good results are important, meaning that FVE may potentially be a substitute of PC imaging, since it contains both a velocity distribution and also velocity map with considerably higher SNR and robustness to partial voluming.

5. Conclusion

In this chapter, was discussed approaches in order to make Fourier Velocity Encoding MRI more suitable for the clinical environment. FVE is a promising MRI technique capable of measuring blood flow in the blood vessels and estimating important biomarkers that are useful for understand and diagnose diseases. It provides a velocity distribution within a voxel instead of a mean velocity map like phase contrast but requires acceleration to be feasible in the clinical setting. So was discussed six different strategies that can reduce drastically the acquisition time. The acceleration techniques discussed are related to the use of variable-density sampling, which may be used along spatial k-space and velocity k-space, partial Fourier acquisition along velocity k-space, temporal acceleration methods such as UNFOLD and k-t BLAST, parallel imaging methods and compressive sensing.

On the other hand, was proposed a novel method for estimating high-resolution velocity maps from low-resolution FVE measurements. This method is based on a PDE-constrained optimization that incorporates the FVE signal model and the Navier-Stokes equation. Results showed that it is possible to obtain highly accurate velocity maps from the FVE distributions. Finally, it can be concluded that FVE datasets can be acquired in time scale comparable to the gold standard phase contrast, it provides more velocity information, since it contains a velocity distribution, and also can provide the actual velocity map as long as a constrained-optimization problem to restore the velocity map is solved.

Author details

Vinicius C. Rispoli*, Joao L.A. Carvalho, Cristiano J. Miosso and Fabiano A. Soares

*Address all correspondence to: vrispoli@pgea.unb.br

University of Brasilia, Brazil

References

[1] Manning WJ, Pennell DJ. Cardiovascular Magnetic Resonance. Elsevier; 2010

[2] Hoskins PR. Accuracy of maximum velocity estimates made using Doppler ultrasound systems. The British Journal of Radiology. 1996;**69**(818):172-177

[3] Winkler AJ, Wu J. Correction of intrinsic spectral broadening errors in Doppler peak velocity measurements made with phased sector and linear array transducers. Ultrasound in Medicine & Biology. 1995;**21**(8):1029-1035

[4] O'Donnell M. NMR blood flow imaging using multiecho, phase contrast sequences. Medical Physics. 1985;**12**(1):59-64

[5] Gonzales E, Carvalho J. Does phase contrast MRI provide the mean velocity of the spins within a voxel?. In: Proc, ISMRM, 22nd Annual Meeting; Milan; 2014. p. 2480

[6] Tang C, Blatter DD, Parker DL. Accuracy of phase-contrast flow measurements in the presence of partial-volume effects. Journal of Magnetic Resonance Imaging. 1993;**3**(2): 377-385

[7] Moran PR. A flow velocity zeugmatographic interlace for NMR imaging in humans. Magnetic Resonance Imaging. 1982;**1**(4):197-203

[8] Macgowan CK, Kellenberger CJ, Detsky JS, Roman K, Yoo S-J. Real-time Fourier velocity encoding: An in vivo evaluation. Journal of Magnetic Resonance Imaging. 2005;**21**:297-304

[9] Carvalho JLA. Velocity-encoded magnetic resonance imaging: Acquisition, reconstruction and applications [PhD thesis]. Department of Electrical Engineering, University of Southern California; 2008

[10] Singer JR. Blood flow rates by nuclear magnetic resonance measurements. Science. 1959; **130**(3389):1652-1653

[11] Hahn EL. Detection of sea-water motion by nuclear precession. Journal of Geophysical Research. 1960;**65**(2):776-777

[12] Moran PR, Moran RA, Karstaedt N. Verification and evaluation of internal flow and motion. True magnetic resonance imaging by the phase gradient modulation method. Radiology. 1985;**154**(2):433-441

[13] Nayler GL, Firmin DN, Longmore DB. Blood flow imaging by cine magnetic resonance. Journal of Computer Assisted Tomography. 1986;**10**(5):715-722

[14] Singer JR, Crooks LE. Nuclear magnetic resonance blood flow measurements in the human brain. Science. 1983;**221**(4611):654-656

[15] van Dijk P. Direct cardiac NMR imaging of heart wall and blood flow velocity. Journal of Computer Assisted Tomography. 1984;**8**(3):429-436

[16] Rebergen SA, van der Wall EE, Doornbos J, de Roos A. Magnetic resonance measurement of velocity and flow: Technique, validation, and cardiovascular applications. American Heart Journal. 1993;**126**(6):1439-1456

[17] Glover GH, Pelc NJ. A rapid-gated cine MRI technique. Magnetic Resonance Annual. 1988;**21**(2):299-333

[18] Tsai C-M, Nishimura DG. Reduced aliasing artifacts using variable-density k-space sampling trajectories. Magnetic Resonance in Medicine. 2000;**43**:452-458

[19] Liu CY, Varadarajan P, Pohost GM, Nayak KS. Real-time color overlay cardiac phase contrast spiral imaging at 3 Tesla. In: Proc., SCMR, 9th Annual Scientific Sessions; Miami; 2006

[20] Carvalho JLA, Nayak KS. Accelerated spiral Fourier velocity encoded imaging. In: Proc, ISMRM, 15th Annual Meeting; Berlin; 2007. p. 588

[21] Carvalho JLA, Nayak KS. Rapid quantitation of cardiovascular flow using slice-selective Fourier velocity encoding with spiral readouts. Magnetic Resonance in Medicine. 2007; **57**(4):639-646

[22] DiCarlo JC, Hargreaves BA, Nayak KS, Hu BS, Pauly JM, Nishimura DG. Variable-density one-shot Fourier velocity encoding. Magnetic Resonance in Medicine. 2005;**54**(3):645-655

[23] Hu BS, Pauly JM, Macovski A. Localized real-time velocity spectra determination. Magnetic Resonance in Medicine. 1993;**30**(3):393-398

[24] Irarrazabal P, Hu BS, Pauly JM, Nishimura DG. Spatially resolved and localized real-time velocity distribution. Magnetic Resonance in Medicine. 1993;**30**(2):207-212

[25] Santos JM, Kerr AB, Lee D, McConnell MV, Yang PC, Hu BS, Pauly JM. Comprehensive valve evaluation system. In: Proc, ISMRM, 15th Annual Meeting; Berlin; 2007. p. 2551

[26] Carvalho JLA, DiCarlo JC, Kerr AB, Nayak KS. Reconstruction of variable-density data in Fourier velocity encoding. In: Proc, ISMRM, 15th Annual Meeting; Berlin; 2007. p. 2514

[27] Noll DC, Nishimura DG, Macovski A. Homodyne detection in magnetic resonance imaging. IEEE Transactions on Medical Imaging. 2001;**10**(2):154-163

[28] Steeden JA, Jones A, Pandya B, Atkinson D, Taylor AM, Muthurangu V. High-resolution slice-selective Fourier velocity encoding in congenital heart disease using spiral SENSE with velocity unwrap. Magnetic Resonance in Medicine. 2012;**67**:1538-1546

[29] Riederer SJ, Tasciyan T, Farzaneh F, Lee JN, Wright RC, Herfkens RJ. MR fluoroscopy: Technical feasibility. Magnetic Resonance in Medicine. 1988;**8**(1):1-15

[30] Madore B, Glover GH, Pelc NJ. Unaliasing by Fourier-encoding the overlaps using the temporal dimension (UNFOLD), applied to cardiac imaging and fMRI. Magnetic Resonance in Medicine. 1999;**42**(5):813-828

[31] Tsao J. On the UNFOLD method. Magnetic Resonance in Medicine. 2002;**47**(1):202-207

[32] Tsao J, Boesiger P, Pruessmann KP. k-t BLAST and k-t SENSE: Dynamic MRI with high frame rate exploiting spatiotemporal correlations. Magnetic Resonance in Medicine. 2003; **50**(5):1031-1042

[33] Macgowan CK, Madore B. Application of UNFOLD to real-time Fourier velocity encoding. In: Proc, ISMRM, 14th Annual Meeting; Seattle; 2006. p. 872

[34] Pruessmann KP, Weiger M, Bornert P, Boesiger P. Advances in sensitivity encoding with arbitrary k-space trajectories. Magnetic Resonance in Medicine. 2001;**46**(4):638-651

[35] Lustig M, Pauly JM. SPIRiT: Iterative self-consistent parallel imaging reconstruction from arbitrary k-space. Magnetic Resonance in Medicine. 2010;**64**:457-471

[36] Lyra-Leite DM, Carvalho JLA. Parallel imaging acceleration of spiral Fourier velocity encoded MRI using SPIRiT. In: Proc 34th International Conference, IEEE Engineering in Medicine and Biology Society; Seattle; 2012. pp. 416-419

[37] Lyra-Leite DM, Nayak KS, Carvalho JLA. Acceleration of spiral Fourier velocity encoded MRI using 3D SPIRiT. In: Proc, ISMRM, 21st Annual Meeting; 2013. p. 1352

[38] Lustig M, Donoho D, Santos J, Pauly J. Compressive sensing MRI. IEEE Signal Processing Magazine. 2008;**25**(2):72-82

[39] Miosso CJ, von Borries R, Pierluissi H. Compressive sensing with prior information: Requirements and probabilities of reconstruction in ℓ_1-minimization. IEEE Transactions on Signal Processing. 2013;**61**(9):2150-2164

[40] Kwak Y, Nam S, Akçakaya M, Basha T, Goddu B, Manning W, Tarokh V, Nezafat R. Accelerated aortic flow assessment with compressed sensing with and without use of the sparsity of the complex difference image. Magnetic Resonance in Medicine. 2013;**70**(3):851-858

[41] Gamper U, Boesiger P, Kozerke S. Compressed sensing in dynamic MRI. Magnetic Resonance in Medicine. 2008;**59**:365-373. DOI: 10.1002/mrm.21477

[42] Hilbert F, Wech T, Hahn D, Köstler H. Accelerated radial Fourier-velocity encoding using compressed sensing. Zeitschrift für Medizinische Physik. 2014;**24**(3):190-200

[43] Baraniuk RG. Compressive sensing [lecture notes]. IEEE Signal Processing Magazine. 2007;**24**:118-121

[44] Donoho DL. Compressive sensing. IEEE Transactions on Information Theory. 2006;**52**(4):1289-1306

[45] Miosso CJ, von Borries R, Argaez M, Velazquez L, Quintero C, Potes CM. Compressive sensing reconstruction with prior information by iteratively reweighted least-squares. IEEE Transactions on Signal Processing. 2009;**57**(6):2424-2431

[46] Miosso CJ. Compressive sensing with prior information applied to magnetic resonance imaging [PhD thesis]. Department of Electrical and Computer Engineering, University of Texas at El Paso; 2010

[47] Candès EJ, Romberg J, Tao T. Stable signal recovery from incomplete and inaccurate measurements. Communications on Pure and Applied Mathematics. 2006;**59**(8):1207-1223

[48] Candès EJ, Romberg J, Tao T. Robust uncertainty principles: Exact signal reconstruction from highly incomplete frequency information. IEEE Transactions on Information Theory. 2006;**52**:489-509

[49] Mousavi A, Patel AB, Baraniuk RG. A deep learning approach to structured signal recovery. In: 53rd Annual Allerton Conference on Communication, Control, and Computing (Allerton); 2015. pp. 1336-1343

[50] Palangi H, Ward R, Deng L. Distributed compressive sensing: A deep learning approach. IEEE Transactions on Signal Processing. 2016;**64**(17):4504-4518

[51] Marinelli L, Khare K, King K, Darrow R, Hardy C. Accelerated 2D Fourier-velocity encoded MRI using compressed sensing. In: Proc, ISMRM, 17th Annual Meeting; 2009. p. 2827

[52] Chorin A, Marsden J. A Mathematical Introduction to Fluid Mechanics. Springer; 2000

[53] Gresho P, Sani R. Incompressible Flow and the Finite Element Method. Wiley; 2000

[54] Carvalho JLA, Nielsen JF, Nayak KS. Feasibility of in vivo measurement of carotid wall shear rate using spiral Fourier velocity encoded MRI. Magnetic Resonance in Medicine. 2010;**63**(6):1537-1547

[55] Rispoli VC, Carvalho JLA. Deriving high-resolution velocity maps from low-resolution Fourier velocity encoded MRI data. In: IEEE 10th International Symposium on Biomedical Imaging; 2013. pp. 334-337

[56] Wang Y, Yang J, Yin W, Zhang Y. A new alternating minimization algorithm for total variation image reconstruction. SIAM Journal on Imaging Sciences. 2008;**1**(3):248-272

Chapter 9

Basics of Chemical Exchange Saturation Transfer (CEST) Magnetic Resonance Imaging

Kenya Murase

Additional information is available at the end of the chapter

http://dx.doi.org/10.5772/intechopen.71645

Abstract

Chemical exchange saturation transfer (CEST) is one of the contrast mechanisms in magnetic resonance imaging (MRI) and has been used to detect dilute proteins through the interaction between bulk water and labile solute protons. Amide proton transfer (APT) MRI has been developed for imaging diseases such as acute stroke. Moreover, various CEST agents have been explored to enhance the CEST effect. The contrast mechanism of CEST or APT MRI, however, is complex and depends not only on the concentration of amide protons or CEST agents and exchange properties, but also varies with imaging parameters such as radiofrequency (RF) power and magnetic field strength. When there are multiple exchangeable pools within a single CEST system, the contrast mechanism of CEST becomes even more complex. Numerical simulations are useful and effective for analyzing the complex contrast mechanism of CEST and for investigating the optimal imaging parameter values. In this chapter, we present the basics of CEST or APT MRI and a simple and fast numerical method for solving the time-dependent Bloch-McConnell equations for analyzing the behavior of magnetization and/or contrast mechanism in CEST or APT MRI. We also present a method for analyzing the behavior of magnetization in spin-locking CEST MRI.

Keywords: Bloch-McConnell equations, numerical solution, chemical exchange saturation transfer (CEST) MRI, amide proton transfer (APT) MRI, spin-locking

1. Introduction

Chemical exchange saturation transfer (CEST) is one of the contrast mechanisms in magnetic resonance imaging (MRI) [1] and has been increasingly used to detect dilute proteins through the interaction between bulk water protons and labile solute protons [2–4]. Amide proton transfer (APT) MRI has been developed for imaging diseases such as acute stroke and cancer, and is now under intensive evaluation for clinical translation [5, 6]. APT MRI is a particular type of CEST MRI that specifically probes labile amide protons of endogenous mobile proteins and peptides in tissue [5, 6]. In addition to APT MRI [5, 6], useful CEST MRI contrast for clinical imaging can be generated from amine protons [7], hydroxyl protons [8], glycosaminoglycans [9], and glutamate [10], as well as from changes in creatine and lactate concentrations [11]. Glucose and iopamidol have been used as exogenous CEST agents that have been administered to patients [12, 13]. Moreover, various CEST agents have been energetically developed to detect the parameters that reflect tissue molecular environment such as hydrogen ion exponent (pH) and/or to enhance the CEST effect [14].

In CEST or APT MRI, the exchangeable proton spins are saturated, and the saturation is transferred upon chemical exchange to the bulk water pool [1, 15]. As a result, a large contrast enhancement in bulk water can be achieved. The contrast mechanism of CEST or APT MRI, however, is complex and depends not only on the concentration of amide protons or CEST agents, relaxation, and exchange properties but also varies with imaging parameters such as radiofrequency (RF) power and magnetic field strength [15]. When there are multiple exchangeable pools within a single CEST system, the contrast mechanism of CEST becomes all the more complex [16]. Numerical simulations are useful and effective for analyzing the complex CEST contrast mechanism and for investigating the optimal imaging parameter values [17, 18]. In order to perform extensive numerical simulations for CEST or APT MRI, it requires the development of a simple and fast numerical method for obtaining the solutions to the time-dependent Bloch-McConnell equations.

In this chapter, we present the basics of CEST or APT MRI and a simple and fast numerical method for solving the time-dependent Bloch-McConnell equations for analyzing the behavior of magnetization and/or contrast mechanism in CEST or APT MRI. We also present it in SL CEST MRI.

2. Bloch-McConnell equations in the presence of CEST

2.1. Two-pool chemical exchange model

A two-pool chemical exchange model is illustrated in **Figure 1**. A and B in **Figure 1** represent the pools of bulk water protons and labile solute protons, respectively. The time-dependent Bloch-McConnell equations for the two-pool chemical exchange model in CEST or APT MRI are expressed as [17, 18].

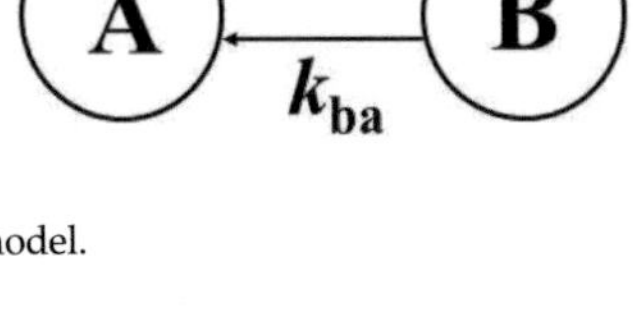

Figure 1. Two-pool chemical exchange model.

http://dx.doi.org/10.5772/intechopen.71645

$$\begin{cases} \dfrac{dM_x^a(t)}{dt} = -R_2^a M_x^a(t) - k_{ab} M_x^a(t) + \Delta\omega_a M_y^a(t) - \omega_1^y M_z^a(t) + k_{ba} M_x^b(t) \\ \dfrac{dM_y^a(t)}{dt} = -\Delta\omega_a M_x^a(t) - R_2^a M_y^a(t) - k_{ab} M_y^a(t) + \omega_1^x M_z^a(t) + k_{ba} M_y^b(t) \\ \dfrac{dM_z^a(t)}{dt} = -\omega_1^y M_x^a(t) - \omega_1^x M_y^a(t) - R_1^a M_z^a(t) - k_{ab} M_z^a(t) + k_{ba} M_z^b(t) + R_1^a M_0^a \\ \dfrac{dM_x^b(t)}{dt} = k_{ab} M_x^a(t) - k_{ba} M_x^a(t) - R_2^b M_x^b(t) + \Delta\omega_b M_y^b(t) - \omega_1^y M_z^b(t) \\ \dfrac{dM_y^b(t)}{dt} = k_{ab} M_y^a(t) - \Delta\omega_b M_x^b(t) - R_2^b M_y^b(t) - k_{ba} M_y^b(t) + \omega_1^x M_z^b(t) \\ \dfrac{dM_z^b(t)}{dt} = k_{ab} M_z^a(t) + \omega_1^y M_y^b(t) - \omega_1^x M_y^b(t) - R_1^b M_z^b(t) - k_{ba} M_z^b(t) + R_1^b M_0^b \end{cases} \quad (1)$$

where superscripts a and b show the parameters in pool A and pool B, respectively. For example, $M_x^a(t)$, $M_y^a(t)$, and $M_z^a(t)$ are the x, y, and z magnetization components in pool A at time t, respectively. R_1^a and R_2^a are the reciprocals of the longitudinal (T_1^a) and transverse relaxation times (T_2^a), that is, the longitudinal and transverse relaxation rates in pool A, respectively. k_{ab} and k_{ba} denote the exchange rate from spins in pool A to those in pool B and that from spins in pool B to those in pool A, respectively (**Figure 1**). M_0^a and M_0^b are the thermal equilibrium z magnetization components in pool A and pool B, respectively. $\Delta\omega_a = \omega_a - \omega$ and $\Delta\omega_b = \omega_b - \omega$, where ω_a, ω_b, and ω denote the Larmor frequencies in pool A and pool B, and the frequency of the RF-pulse irradiation, respectively. ω_1^x and ω_1^y are the x and y components of the amplitude of the RF-pulse irradiation (ω_1), respectively. Note that $\omega_1 = \gamma B_1$, where γ and B_1 are the gyromagnetic ratio ($\gamma/2\pi = 42.58$ MH$_z$/T) and RF power, respectively. When the RF pulse is applied along an angle φ from the x-axis of the rotating frame as illustrated in **Figure 2**, ω_1^x and ω_1^y are represented by $\omega_1^x = \omega_1 \cos\phi$ and $\omega_1^y = \omega_1 \sin\phi$, respectively. When the RF pulse is applied along the x-axis of the rotating frame, ω_1^x and ω_1^y become ω_1 and 0, respectively.

The differential equations given by Eq. (1) can be combined into one vector equation (homogeneous linear differential equation) [18]:

$$\frac{d\mathbf{M}(t)}{dt} = \mathbf{A}(\omega, \omega_1, \phi) \cdot \mathbf{M}(t), \quad (2)$$

where

$$\mathbf{M}(t) = \left[M_x^a(t) \;\; M_y^a(t) \;\; M_z^a(t) \;\; M_x^b(t) \;\; M_y^b(t) \;\; M_z^b(t) \;\; \mathbf{1} \right]^T \quad (3)$$

and

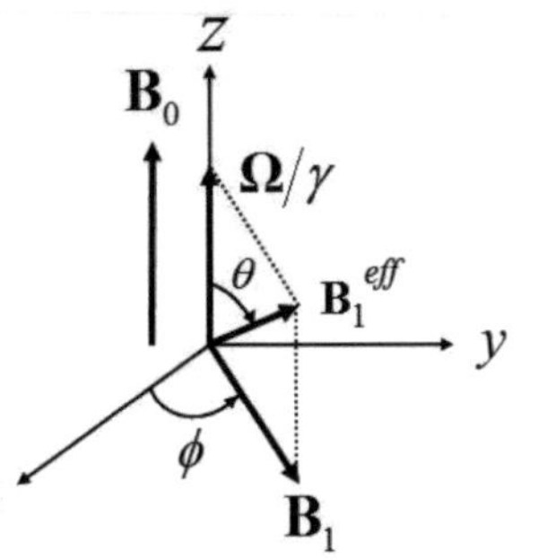

Figure 2. Parameters for analyzing the behavior of magnetization in the rotating frame.

$$\mathbf{A}(\omega,\omega_1,\phi)=\begin{bmatrix} -(R_2^a+k_{ab}) & \Delta\omega_a & -\omega_1^y & k_{ba} & 0 & 0 & 0 \\ -\Delta\omega_a & -(R_2^a+k_{ab}) & \omega_1^x & 0 & k_{ba} & 0 & 0 \\ \omega_1^y & -\omega_1^x & -(R_1^a+k_{ab}) & 0 & 0 & k_{ba} & R_1^a M_0^a \\ k_{ab} & 0 & 0 & -(R_2^b+k_{ba}) & \Delta\omega_b & -\omega_1^y & 0 \\ 0 & k_{ab} & 0 & -\Delta\omega_b & -(R_2^b+k_{ba}) & \omega_1^x & 0 \\ 0 & 0 & k_{ab} & \omega_1^y & -\omega_1^x & -(R_1^b+k_{ba}) & R_1^b M_0^b \\ 0 & 0 & 0 & 0 & 0 & 0 & 0 \end{bmatrix}. \tag{4}$$

T in Eq. (3) denotes the matrix transpose.

For simplicity, we assume that the RF pulse is applied along the x-axis of the rotating frame, that is, $\phi=0$. According to Koss et al. [19], the matrix $\mathbf{A}(\omega,\omega_1,0)$ can be given by.

$$\mathbf{A}(\omega,\omega_1,0)=\begin{bmatrix} \mathbf{E} & \mathbf{C} \\ \mathbf{0} & \mathbf{0} \end{bmatrix}, \tag{5}$$

where **E** is the evolution matrix and **C** is the constant-term matrix. Furthermore, **E** is given by.

$$\mathbf{E}=\mathbf{R}+\mathbf{K}. \tag{6}$$

In the case of **A** given by Eq. (4), **R** is reduced to.

$$\mathbf{R}=\begin{bmatrix} \mathbf{R^a} & \mathbf{0} \\ \mathbf{0} & \mathbf{R^b} \end{bmatrix}, \tag{7}$$

where

$$\mathbf{R}^a=\begin{bmatrix} -R_2^a & \Delta\omega_a & 0 \\ -\Delta\omega_a & -R_2^a & \omega_1 \\ 0 & -\omega_1 & R_1^a \end{bmatrix}, \tag{8}$$

and

http://dx.doi.org/10.5772/intechopen.71645

$$\mathbf{R}^b = \begin{bmatrix} -R_2^b & \Delta\omega_b & 0 \\ -\Delta\omega_b & -R_2^b & \omega_1 \\ 0 & -\omega_1 & R_1^b \end{bmatrix}, \tag{9}$$

K in Eq. (6) is given by

$$\mathbf{K} = \begin{bmatrix} -k_{ab} & k_{ba} \\ k_{ab} & -k_{ba} \end{bmatrix} \otimes \mathbf{I}, \tag{10}$$

where **I** is a 3-by-3 identity matrix and ⊗ denotes the Kronecker tensor product. **C** in Eq. (5) is given by.

$$\mathbf{C} = \begin{bmatrix} R_1^a M_0^a & R_1^b M_0^b \end{bmatrix}^T \otimes \begin{bmatrix} \mathbf{0} & \mathbf{0} & \mathbf{1} \end{bmatrix}^{\mathrm{T}}. \tag{11}$$

The solution of Eq. (2) with ϕ being 0 can be given by [18].

$$\mathbf{M}(t) = e^{\mathbf{A}(\omega,\omega_1,0)t}\mathbf{M}(0), \tag{12}$$

where t represents the so-called saturation time and $\mathbf{M}(0)$ is the matrix of initial values at $t=0$. $e^{\mathbf{A}(\omega,\,\omega_1,\,0)t}$ is the matrix exponential.

It should be noted that mass balance imposes the following relationship between the exchange rates (k_{ab} and k_{ba}) of pool A and pool B [17]:

$$k_{ab} = (k_{ab} + k_{ba})\cdot\frac{M_0^b}{M_0^a + M_0^b} \tag{13}$$

and

$$k_{ba} = (k_{ab} + k_{ba})\cdot\frac{M_0^a}{M_0^a + M_0^b} \tag{14}$$

2.2. Three-pool chemical exchange model

Figure 3 illustrates a three-pool chemical exchange model in which pool a represents the bulk water pool. In this case, **R** and **K** are given by [19].

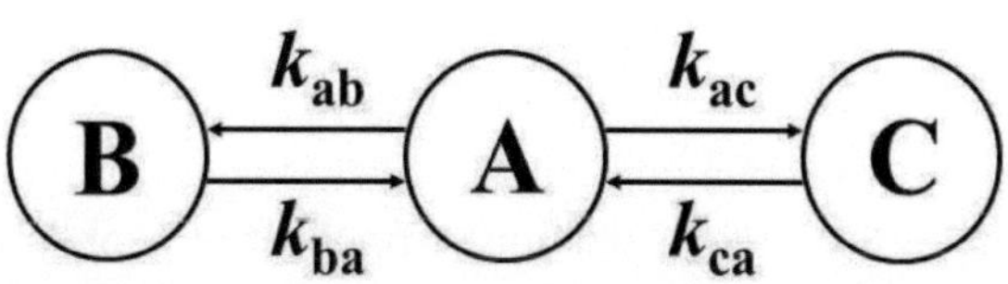

Figure 3. Three pool chemical exchange model.

$$\mathbf{R} = \begin{bmatrix} \boldsymbol{R}^a & 0 & 0 \\ 0 & \boldsymbol{R}^b & 0 \\ 0 & 0 & \boldsymbol{R}^c \end{bmatrix} \tag{15}$$

and

$$\mathbf{K} = \begin{bmatrix} -k_{ab} - k_{ac} & k_{ba} & k_{ca} \\ k_{ab} & -k_{ba} & 0 \\ k_{ac} & 0 & -k_{ac} \end{bmatrix} \otimes \mathbf{I}, \tag{16}$$

respectively. $\mathbf{R}^c$ in Eq. (15) is given by Eq. (8) in which the subscript a and superscript a are replaced by c. $\mathbf{C}$ is given by.

$$\mathbf{C} = \left[R_1^a M_0^a \quad R_1^b M_0^b \quad R_1^c M_0^c\right]^T \otimes [\mathbf{0} \quad \mathbf{0} \quad \mathbf{1}]^T. \tag{17}$$

The solutions of other multi-pool chemical exchange models such as an hour-pool chemical exchange model are described in Ref. [20].

2.3. Calculation of Z-spectrum, MTR$_{\text{asym}}$, and PTR

The CEST effect has usually been analyzed using the so-called Z-spectrum [18]. The Z-spectrum is given by the following equation:

$$\text{Z} - \text{spectrum} = \frac{M_z^a(\Delta\omega_{off})}{M_0^a}, \tag{18}$$

where $M_z^a(\Delta\omega_{off})$ is the z magnetization component of bulk water protons (pool A) at $\Delta\omega_{off}$. Note that $\Delta\omega_{off} = -\Delta\omega_a$.

The magnetization transfer asymmetry (MTR$_{\text{asym}}$) analysis has been performed using the following equation [18]:

$$\text{MTR}_{\text{asym}} = \frac{M_z^a(-\Delta\omega_{off}) - M_z^a(\Delta\omega_{off})}{M_0^a}. \tag{19}$$

Instead of MTR$_{\text{asym}}$, the following equation for proton transfer ratio (PTR) has also been used for analyzing the CEST effect [18]:

$$\text{PTR} = \frac{M_z^a(-\Delta\omega_{off}) - M_z^a(\Delta\omega_{off})}{M_z^a(-\Delta\omega_{off})}, \tag{20}$$

where $M_z^a(-\Delta\omega_{off})$ denotes the z magnetization component of pool A at the opposite side of the water resonance ($\Delta\omega_{off}$).

Figure 4(a) shows Z-spectra as a function of offset frequency ($\Delta\omega_{off}$) for various saturation times (0.5, 1, 2, 5, and 10 s) in the two-pool chemical exchange model (**Figure 1**). **Figure 4(b)** shows Z-spectra as a function of $\Delta\omega_{off}$ for various ω_1 values (25, 50, 100, 150, and 200 Hz). It should be noted that because $B_1 = \omega_1/\gamma$, ω_1 values of 25, 50, 100, 150, and 200 Hz correspond to B_1 values of 0.59, 1.17, 2.35, 3.52, and 4.70 μT, respectively. **Figure 4(c)** shows Z-spectra as a function of $\Delta\omega_{off}$ for various M_0^b/M_0^a values (1/500, 1/250, 1/125, 1/100, and 1/50).

In the above simulations, we assumed that T_1^a and T_2^a were 3 s and 100 ms, respectively, and $T_1^b = 1$ s and $T_2^b = 15$ ms [16]. The chemical shift of protons in pool B was set to be 4 ppm. It should be noted that the chemical shift of 4 ppm corresponds to $\Delta\omega_{off}$ of 1192.8 Hz for the magnetic field strength of 7 T. Unless otherwise indicated, $k_{ab} + k_{ba}$ was assumed to be 100 Hz. M_0^a and M_0^b were assumed to be 1 and 1/250, respectively. The saturation time and ω_1 were taken as 2 s and 100 Hz, respectively. The matrix exponential and Kronecker tensor product were calculated using the MATLAB® functions "expm" and "kron," respectively.

The peaks at 0 Hz (0 ppm) and 1192.8 Hz (4 ppm) in **Figure 4** derived from pool A and pool B, respectively. As shown in **Figure 4(a)** and **Figure 4(b)**, Z-spectra changed largely depending on the saturation time and ω_1, that is, Z-spectra became broad and tended to saturate with increasing saturation time and ω_1. As shown in **Figure 4(c)**, the peaks at 1192.8 Hz increased with increasing M_0^b/M_0^a value.

Figure 5 shows cases for the three-pool chemical exchange model (**Figure 3**) consisting of bulk water (pool A) and two labile proton pools (pool B and pool C). In these cases, we assumed that $T_1^a = 3$ s, $T_2^a = 100$ *ms*, $T_1^b = T_1^c = 1$ s, and $T_2^b = T_2^c = 15$ ms [16]. The chemical shifts of two labile proton pools were set to be 4 ppm ($\Delta\omega_{off}$=1192.8 Hz for the magnetic field strength of 7 T) and 5 ppm ($\Delta\omega_{off}$=1491.0 Hz for 7 T). Unless otherwise indicated, $k_{ab} + k_{ba}$, $k_{ac} + k_{ca}$, and $k_{bc} + k_{cb}$ were assumed to be 100 Hz, 300 Hz, and 100 Hz, respectively. M_0^a, M_0^b, and M_0^c were assumed to be 1, 1/250, and 1/500, respectively. The saturation time and ω_1 were taken as 5 s and 50 Hz, respectively.

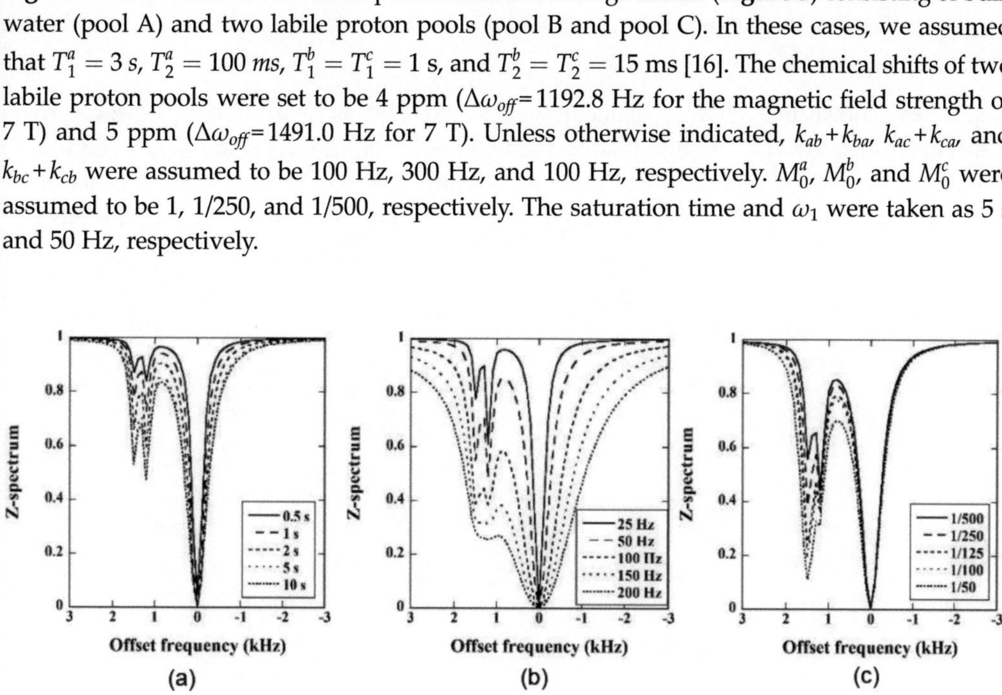

Figure 4. Z-spectra as a function of $\Delta\omega_{off}$ for various values of saturation time (a), ω_1 (b), and M_0^b/M_0^a (c) in the two-pool chemical exchange model.

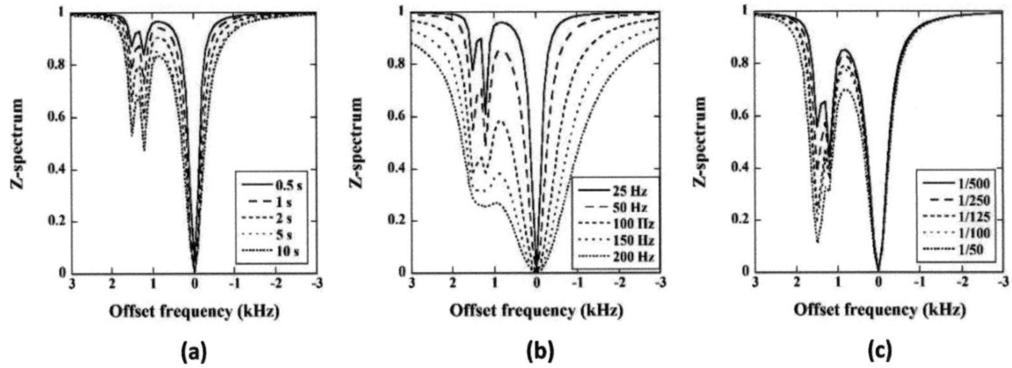

Figure 5. Z-spectra as a function of $\Delta\omega_{off}$ for various values of saturation time (a), ω_1 (b), and M_0^c/M_0^a (c) in the three-pool chemical exchange model.

Figure 5(a) shows Z-spectra as a function of $\Delta\omega_{off}$ for various saturation times (0.5, 1, 2, 5, and 10 s). The peaks at 0 Hz (0 ppm), 1192.8 Hz (4 ppm), and 1491.0 Hz (5 ppm) derive from pool A, pool B, and pool C, respectively. As shown in **Figure 5(a)**, Z-spectra changed largely depending on the saturation time, that is, Z-spectra became broad and tended to saturate with increasing saturation time. **Figure 5(b)** shows Z-spectra as a function of $\Delta\omega_{off}$ for various ω_1 values (25, 50, 100, 150, and 200 Hz). As in **Figure 4(b)**, Z-spectra became broad with increasing ω_1 value. **Figure 5(c)** shows Z-spectra as a function of $\Delta\omega_{off}$ for various M_0^c/M_0^a values (1/500, 1/250, 1/125, 1/100, and 1/50). The peaks at 1491.0 Hz increased with increasing M_0^c/M_0^a value.

Figure 6(a) shows the MTR_{asym} values given by Eq. (19) as a function of ω_1 for various saturation times (0.5, 1, 2, 5, and 10 s) in the two-pool chemical exchange model (**Figure 1**), whereas **Figure 6(b)** shows those as a function of saturation time for various ω_1 values (25, 50, 100, 150, and 200 Hz). As shown in **Figure 6(a)**, when ω_1 was small, MTR_{asym} tended to

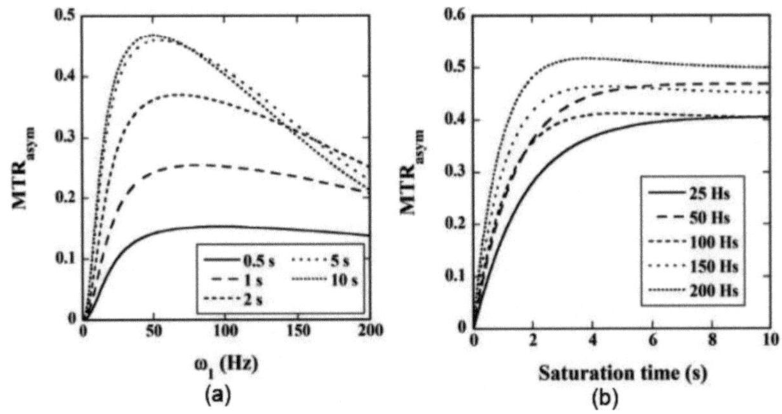

Figure 6. (a) MTR_{asym} values as a function of ω_1 for various saturation times in the two – pool chemical exchange model. (b) MTRasym values as a function of saturation time for various ω_1 values.

http://dx.doi.org/10.5772/intechopen.71645

increase with increasing ω_1 and saturation time. However, when ω_1 was large, MTR_{asym} tended to saturate or decrease with increasing ω_1 value, depending on the saturation time. As shown in **Figure 6(b)**, MTR_{asym} tended to saturate with increasing saturation time for all ω_1 values.

Figure 7(a) shows the PTR values given by Eq. (20) as a function of ω_1 for various saturation times (0.5, 1, 2, 5, and 10 s) in the two-pool chemical exchange model (**Figure 1**), whereas **Figure 7(b)** shows those as a function of saturation time for various ω_1 values (25, 50, 100, 150, and 200 Hz). As shown in **Figure 7**, although PTR showed almost the same tendency with MTR_{asym} (**Figure 6**), the change in the PTR value depending on the saturation time or ω_1 was larger than that in the MTR_{asym} value.

In this study, we presented a simple equation for solving the time-dependent Bloch-McConnell equations, in which our previous method [18] and the approach presented by Koss et al. [19] were combined. Our method can be easily expanded to multi-pool chemical exchange models by modifying the matrix **A** in Eq. (2). We previously reported that the solutions obtained by our method agreed with the analytical solutions given by Mulkern and Williams, [21] and the numerical solutions obtained using a fourth/fifth-order Runge–Kutta-Fehlberg (RKF) algorithm [18], indicating the validity of our method. In addition, our method considerably reduced the computation time as compared with the RKF algorithm [18]. These results suggest that our method will be useful in calculating the parameters such as the exchange rate of CEST agents using the non-linear least-squares fitting method [17].

As previously described, the so-called Z-spectrum has usually been used to analyze the CEST effect [18]. The Z-spectrum is obtained by plotting the z magnetization component of bulk water protons (M_z^a) in the form of M_z^a versus $\Delta\omega_{off}$ [Eq. (18)]. **Figure 4(a)** and **Figure 5(a)** showed that the saturation time affected the Z-spectra, and the CEST effect increased and saturated with increasing saturation time. The fact that the CEST effect saturates with increasing saturation time is more clearly confirmed by the relationship between MTR_{asym} or PTR,

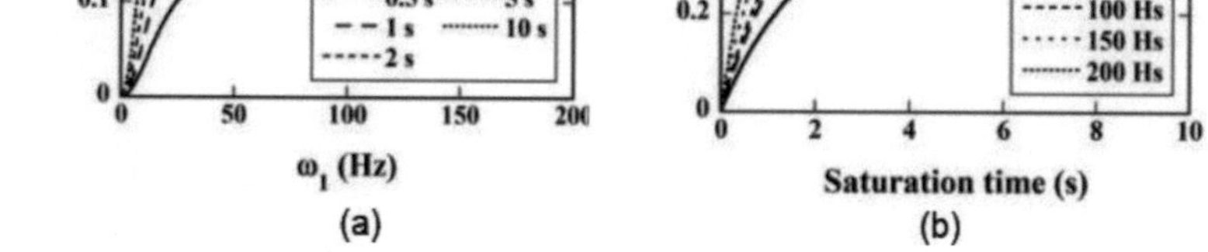

Figure 7. (a) PTR values as a function of ω_1 for various saturation times in the two − pool chemical exchange model. (b) PTR values as a function of saturation time for various ω_1 values.

and the saturation time shown in **Figure 6(b)** or **Figure 7(b)**. As shown in **Figure 4(b)** and **Figure 5(b)**, ω_1 also affected the Z-spectra. Although the CEST effect increased with increasing ω_1 value, the separation among peaks in the Z-spectrum plots degraded with increasing ω_1 value. The influence of ω_1 on the CEST effect is also clearly demonstrated by the relationship between MTR_{asym} and PTR, and ω_1 shown in **Figure 6(a)** or **Figure 7(a)**. The use of large ω_1 may directly saturate bulk water protons, causing the so-called spillover effect [18]. The results shown in **Figures 4–7** suggest that the values of imaging parameters in CEST MRI such as the saturation time and ω_1 must be determined in consideration of both the CEST effect and spillover effect. Our method is useful for determining the optimal values of imaging parameters in CEST MRI.

2.4. Calculation of $R_{1\rho}$ and $R_{2\rho}$

The longitudinal relaxation rate in the rotating frame ($R_{1\rho}$) can be obtained from the negative of the largest (least negative) real eigenvalue (λ_1) of the matrix **A** in Eq. (2), that is, $R_{1\rho} = -\lambda_1$ [19, 22].

The transverse relaxation rate in the rotating frame ($R_{2\rho}$) can be obtained from the absolute value of the largest real part of the complex eigenvalue (λ_2) of the matrix **A** in Eq. (2), that is, $R_{2\rho} = |\mathrm{Re}(\lambda_2)|$ [22], where Re denotes the real part of a complex number.

Figure 8 shows the common logarithm of $R_{1\rho}$ (a) and $R_{2\rho}$ (b) as a function of $\Delta\omega_{off}$ for saturation times of 0.5, 1, 2, 5, and 10 s in the two-pool chemical exchange model (**Figure 1**). The peaks at 0 Hz (0 ppm) and 1192.8 Hz (4 ppm) derive from pool A and pool B, respectively. As shown in **Figure 8**, $R_{1\rho}$ and $R_{2\rho}$ were not affected by the saturation time.

Figure 9 shows the common logarithm of $R_{1\rho}$ (a) and $R_{2\rho}$ (b) as a function of $\Delta\omega_{off}$ for ω_1 values of 25, 50, 100, 150, and 200 Hz in the two-pool chemical exchange model (**Figure 1**). As shown in **Figure 9**, both parameters became broad with increasing ω_1 value.

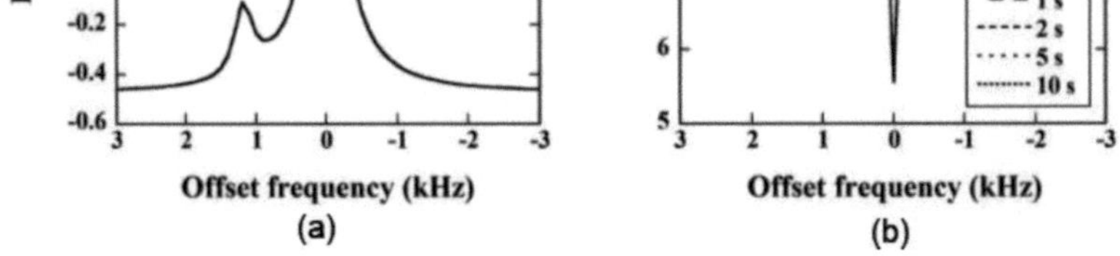

Figure 8. (a) Common logarithm of $R_{1\rho}$ and (b) $R_{2\rho}$ values as a function of $\Delta\omega_{off}$ for various saturation times in the two-pool chemical exchange model.

http://dx.doi.org/10.5772/intechopen.71645

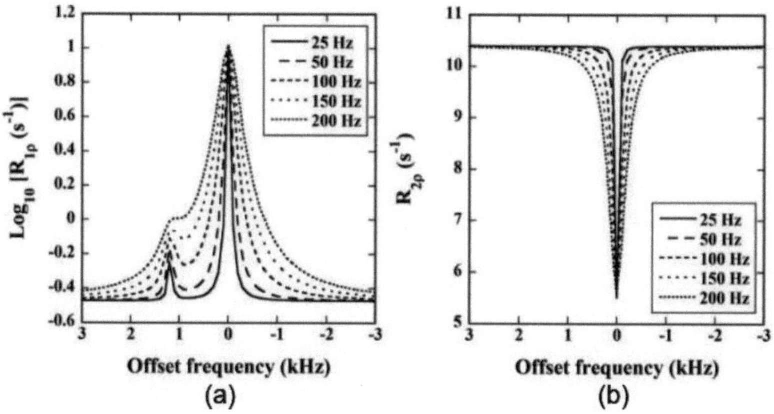

Figure 9. (a) Common logarithm of $R_{1\rho}$ and (b) $R_{2\rho}$ values as a function of $\Delta\omega_{off}$ for various ω_1 values in the two-pool chemical exchange model.

As described above, $R_{1\rho}$ and $R_{2\rho}$ can be obtained from the negative of the largest (least negative) real eigenvalue and the absolute value of the largest real part of the complex eigenvalue of the matrix **A** in Eq. (2), respectively. We previously reported that there was good agreement between the $R_{1\rho}$ and $R_{2\rho}$ values thus obtained and those obtained numerically [22]. These results appear to indicate the validity of these procedures.

As shown in **Figure 8**, $R_{1\rho}$ and $R_{2\rho}$ were not affected by the saturation time, because the matrix **A** in Eq. (2) is independent of the saturation time. When ω_1 was varied, the influence of ω_1 on $R_{1\rho}$ and $R_{2\rho}$ increased with increasing ω_1 value (**Figure 9**). Especially, the separation between peaks in the $R_{1\rho}$ plots degraded with increasing ω_1 value [**Figure 9(a)**]. This also appears to be due to the spillover effect.

3. Spin-locking CEST MRI

3.1. Principle of spin-locking

Longitudinal relaxation time in the rotating frame ($T_{1\rho}$) has been demonstrated to be effective for probing the slow-motion interactions between motion-restricted water molecules and their local macromolecular environment [23] and provides novel image contrast that is not available from conventional MRI techniques. The imaging of biologic tissue based on $T_{1\rho}$ is currently being investigated for various tissues, including articular cartilage, breast, and head and neck [24–26]. In $T_{1\rho}$-weighted MRI of tissues, the image is sensitive to molecular processes that occur over a range of frequencies determined by the amplitude of an applied SL pulse [23].

As pointed out by Jin et al. [27], the SL approach is useful for improving the signal-to-noise ratio (SNR) in CEST MRI. Furthermore, Kogan et al. [28] demonstrated that a combination of the CEST and SL approaches is useful for detecting proton exchange in the slow-to intermediate-exchange regimes.

As earlier described, the Bloch-McConnell equations for the two-pool chemical exchange model (**Figure 1**) in the rotating frame with the same frequency as that of the RF-pulse irradiation is given by Eq. (2) [18, 29]. The solution of Eq. (2) can be given by [18]

$$\mathbf{M}(t) = e^{\mathbf{A}(\omega,\omega_1,\phi)t}\mathbf{M}(0). \tag{21}$$

Figure 10 illustrates the image of the pulse sequence with SL. We assume that the SL pulse (frequency: ω, amplitude: ω_1, and frequency offset: Ω) is applied on the x-axis (**Figure 2**). The effective magnetic field (B_1^{eff}) and its angle with respect to the z – axis (θ) are given by $B_1^{eff} = \sqrt{\omega_1^2 + \Omega^2}/\gamma$ and $\theta = \tan^{-1}(\omega_1/\Omega)$, respectively (**Figure 2**). To achieve SL, the magnetization is first flipped by the θ-degree RF pulse (frequency: ω and amplitude: ω_1^θ) to the x-z plane, then spin locked by B_1^{eff} for a duration of t_{SL}, and then flipped back to the z-axis for imaging (**Figure 10**). The θ-degree RF pulse for flipping is applied on the –y axis, that is, $\phi = -\pi/2$, whereas the θ-degree RF pulse for flipping back is applied on the y axis, that is, $\phi = \pi/2$. The θ-degree rotation matrix for flipping [$\mathbf{R}(\theta)$] is given by [30].

$$\mathbf{R}(\theta) = e^{\mathbf{A}\left(\omega_a,\omega_1^\theta,-\pi/2\right)t_\theta}, \tag{22}$$

where ω_1^θ and t_θ denote the amplitude and the duration of the θ-degree RF-pulse irradiation, respectively (**Figure 10**), and $\omega_1^\theta \times t_\theta = \theta$. Thus, we obtain the magnetization vector immediately after SL for a duration of t_{SL} [$\mathbf{M}^-(t_{SL})$] as.

$$\mathbf{M}^-(t_{SL}) = e^{\mathbf{A}(\omega,\omega_1,0)t_{SL}}\mathbf{R}(\theta)\mathbf{M}(0). \tag{23}$$

The θ-degree rotation matrix for flipping back to the z-axis [$\mathbf{R}(-\theta)$] is given by.

$$\mathbf{R}(-\theta) = e^{\mathbf{A}\left(\omega_a,\omega_1^\theta,\pi/2\right)t_\theta}, \tag{24}$$

Thus, the magnetization vector after flipping back to the z-axis [$\mathbf{M}^+(t_{SL})$] is given by.

$$\mathbf{M}^+(t_{SL}) = \mathbf{R}(-\theta)\mathbf{M}^-(t_{SL}) = \mathbf{R}(-\theta)e^{\mathbf{A}(\omega,\omega_1,0)t_{SL}}\mathbf{R}(\theta)\mathbf{M}(0). \tag{25}$$

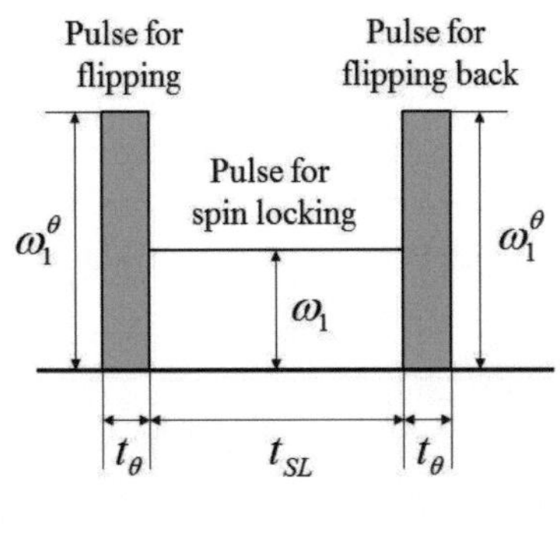

Figure 10. Diagram of spin-locking pulse sequence.

Note that Ω and θ are taken to be 0 and $\pi/2$, respectively, for an on-resonance SL sequence, whereas the saturation pulse is applied without flipping the magnetization in the sequence without SL such as the conventional CEST sequence [15]. Therefore, the magnetization vector after the saturation pulse [$\mathbf{M}(t_{SAT})$] in the conventional CEST MRI is simply expressed as.

$$\mathbf{M}(t_{SAT}) = e^{\mathbf{A}(\omega,\omega_1,0)t_{SAT}}\mathbf{M}(0), \tag{26}$$

where t_{SAT} denotes the duration of saturation.

3.2. Calculation of $T_{1\rho}$

$T_{1\rho}$ can be obtained numerically by fitting the z component of magnetization for t_{SL} [$\mathbf{M}^{+}(t_{SL})$ given by Eq. (25)] in pool A [$M_z^a(t_{SL})$] to the following equation [30]:

$$M_z^a(t_{SL}) = \left(M_0^a - M_{zss}^a\right)e^{-t_{SL}/T_{1\rho}} + M_{zss}^a, \tag{27}$$

where M_{zss}^a denotes the steady-state z component of magnetization in pool A. In this study, we used the Simplex method [31] to calculate $T_{1\rho}$ from Eq. (27).

The approximate solution for $T_{1\rho}$ has been derived by Trott and Palmer [29]:

$$T_{1\rho} \approx \frac{1}{R_1\cos^2\theta + (R_2 + R_{ex})\sin^2\theta}, \tag{28}$$

where $\theta = \tan^{-1}(\omega_1/\Omega)$, $R_{ex} = P_aP_b\Delta\omega^2k_{ex}/\left(\omega_{ae}^2\omega_{be}^2/\omega_e^2 + k_{ex}^2\right)$, $\omega_{ae} = \sqrt{\omega_1^2 + \Delta\omega_a^2}$, $\omega_{be} = \sqrt{\omega_1^2 + \Delta\omega_b^2}$, $\omega_e = \sqrt{\omega_1^2 + \Omega^2}$, $\Omega = \overline{\omega} - \omega$, $\overline{\omega} = P_a\omega_a + P_b\omega_b$, $\Delta\omega = \Delta\omega_b - \Delta\omega_a = \omega_b - \omega_a$, and $k_{ex} = k_{ab} + k_{ba}$. P_a and P_b are the fractional sizes of pool A and pool B, and are given by $P_a = M_0^a/\left(M_0^a + M_0^b\right)$ and $P_b = M_0^b/\left(M_0^a + M_0^b\right)$, respectively. R_1 and R_2 are the population-averaged relaxation rates, and are given by $R_1 = P_aR_1^a + P_bR_1^b$ and $R_2 = P_aR_2^a + P_bR_2^b$, respectively. It should be noted that Ω is the population-averaged offset frequency in this case. M_{zss}^a in Eq. (27) is approximated by [27].

$$\frac{M_{zss}^a}{M_0^a} \approx \frac{R_1\cos^2\theta}{R_{1\rho}}. \tag{29}$$

Figure 11 shows an example of the three-dimensional plots of the magnetization vector in pool A in the two-pool chemical exchange model (**Figure 1**). **Figure 11(a)** and **11(b)** show cases without and with SL, respectively. In these cases, the relaxation time constants were assumed to be $T_1^a = 1.5$ s, $T_2^a = 0.06$ s, $T_1^b = 0.77$ s, and $T_2^b = 0.033$ s [32]. t_θ in Eq. (22) and (24) was taken as 200 μs [27]. ω_1^θ in Eq. (22) and (24) was calculated from $\omega_1^\theta = \theta/t_\theta$. Unless specifically stated, $\Delta\omega$ ($=\omega_b - \omega_a$) and ω_1 were assumed to be 2400 and 1000 Hz, respectively. Ω was assumed to be 2000 Hz. Thus, θ was $\tan^{-1}(\omega_1/\Omega) = \tan^{-1}(1000/2000) \approx 26.6$ degrees. k_{ex} ($=k_{ab} + k_{ba}$) was assumed to be 1500 Hz, and k_{ab} was assumed to be given by $k_{ab} = \left(M_0^b/M_0^a\right)k_{ba}$ [18]. M_0^b/M_0^a was assumed to be 0.03. As shown in **Figure 11(a)**, when the SL pulse was not applied, the magnetization vector rotated largely around B_1^{eff}. On the other hand, when the SL pulse was

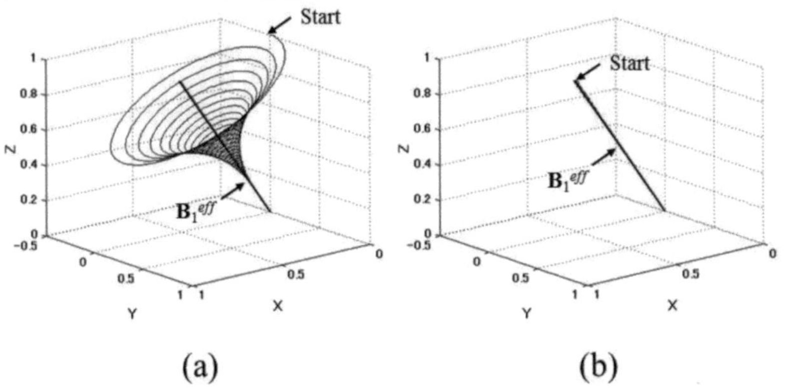

Figure 11. Three-dimensional plots of the magnetization vector in pool A in the two-pool chemical exchange model. (a) and (b) show cases without and with spin-locking pulse, respectively.

applied [**Figure 11(b)**], the magnetization vector moved along B_1^{eff}, and the rotation around B_1^{eff} was suppressed.

When M_0^b/M_0^a was 0.003, there was good agreement between the $T_{1\rho}$ values calculated from Eq. (27) and Trott and Palmer's solutions given by Eq. (28) (data not shown). When M_0^b/M_0^a was 0.03, some difference was observed between them in the off-resonance case. When M_0^b/M_0^a was 0.3, large differences were observed between them in both the on- and off-resonance cases [30].

In this study, we developed a simple and fast method for calculating the magnetization vector in SL CEST MRI, in which a simple matrix equation was derived for solving the time-dependent Bloch-McConnell equations in SL MRI [Eq. (25)] and the θ-degree rotation matrix [Eq. (22)] was introduced for considering the effect of the θ-degree RF pulse for flipping the magnetization. As shown in **Figure 11**, the trajectory of the magnetization vector in the sequence with SL could be visualized by calculating $\mathbf{M}^{-}(t_{SL})$ using Eq. (23), whereas that in the sequence without SL could be visualized by calculating $\mathbf{M}(t_{SAT})$ using Eq. (26). Although **Figure 11** shows the three-dimensional plots observed from one direction, we can observe the trajectory of the magnetization vector from various directions by rotating the plot. If we compared the three-dimensional plots with and without SL (**Figure 11**), then the effect of SL is well understood. Therefore, our method is helpful for visually understanding the effect of SL. In addition, as our method allows us to simply and quickly calculate the time evolution of the magnetization vector under various study conditions in SL CEST MRI, our method can also be useful for optimizing the study conditions in SL CEST MRI.

As previously described, when M_0^b/M_0^a was small, that is, when the population of two pools was highly asymmetric, the $T_{1\rho}$ values calculated from Eq. (27) agreed with the solutions given by Eq. (28). However, the difference between them increased with increasing M_0^b/M_0^a [30]. This finding appears to be due to the fact that Trott and Palmer's solution [Eq. (28)] was derived by approximating the parameters such as relaxation rates using their population-averaged values, and thus the validity of this approximation decreases with decreasing asymmetry in the populations of the two pools.

Although we treated the two-pool chemical exchange model (**Figure 1**) for analyzing $T_{1\rho}$ or $R_{1\rho}$ in SL CEST MRI, recent investigations have shown the importance of improved theoretical approaches for describing multi-site chemical exchange phenomena [33, 34]. Thus, Trott and Palmer [33] have tried to generalize their approach for $T_{1\rho}$ or $R_{1\rho}$ [29]. For such purposes, it is necessary to expand the Bloch-McConnell equations to those based on multi-pool chemical exchange models. Our method can be easily expanded to multi-pool chemical exchange models by modifying the matrix **A** given by Eq. (4) [20] as previously described, and it is helpful for testing the validity of newly developed approaches for analyzing multi-site chemical exchange phenomena.

4. Correction of B_0 and B_1

As previously described, the CEST effect has usually been analyzed using MTR_{asym} [Eq. (19)] or PTR [Eq. (20)]. However, these parameters are susceptible to the B_0 inhomogeneity of the static magnetic field. When there exists the B_0 inhomogeneity, the spillover effect is no longer symmetric. Furthermore, the B_1 inhomogeneity of the RF pulse may also cause spatial variation in labeling efficiency and spillover factor [35]. Apart from the efforts in improving magnetic field inhomogeneities using hardware-based methods, such as parallel transmit technologies [36], post-processing algorithms have been developed for field inhomogeneity correction [37, 38].

Kim et al. [37] showed that direct water saturation imaging allows measurement of the absolute water frequency in each voxel, allowing proper centering of Z-spectra on a voxel-by-voxel basis independent of spatial B_0 field variations, and that the B_0 inhomogeneity in CEST MRI can be corrected on a voxel-by-voxel basis through the centering of Z-spectra. This method is called "water saturation shift referencing (WASSR)" approach. This method, however, would require acquisition of saturation images at 20–40 frequencies [38]. Since the SNR of CEST MRI is low, multiple acquisitions for each frequency offset of complete Z-spectra would be needed, which is not practical in the clinical setting. Zhou et al. demonstrated that a practical six-offset multi-acquisition method combined with a single reference Z-spectrum to acquire high-SNR CEST MRI can accomplish improved CEST MRI with B_0 inhomogeneity correction within an acceptable scanning time [38].

A B_1-correction of CEST contrasts is crucial for the evaluation of data obtained in clinical studies at high field strengths with strong B_1-inhomogeneities. To correct for the B_1 inhomogeneity, a B_1 map is acquired for correction of Z-spectra using either a calibration [39] or an interpolation approach [40]. Singh et al. [39] developed an approach for B_1 inhomogeneity correction based on acquiring calibration data at a coarsely sampled B_1 values in conjunction with the measured B_1 maps, whereas Windschuh et al. [40] developed an approach based on Lorentzian line fits.

The comprehensive methods like simultaneous mapping of B_0 and B_1 fields [35, 41], and model-based correction algorithm, [42] have also been developed to improve the accuracy of MTR_{asym} or PTR.

Acknowledgements

This work was supported, in part, by a Grant-in-Aid for Challenging Exploratory Research (Grant No. 25670532) from the Japan Society for the Promotion of Science.

Author details

Kenya Murase

Address all correspondence to: murase@sahs.med.osaka-u.ac.jp

Department of Medical Physics and Engineering, Division of Medical Technology and Science, Faculty of Health Science, Graduate School of Medicine, Osaka University, Osaka, Japan

References

[1] Ward K, Aletras A, Balaban R. A new class of contrast agents for MRI based on proton chemical exchange dependent saturation transfer (CEST). Journal of Magnetic Resonance. 2000;**143**:79-87

[2] Goffeney N, Bulte JWM, Duyn J, Bryant LH, van Zijl PCM. Sensitive NMR detection of cationic-polymer-based gene delivery systems using saturation transfer via proton exchange. Journal of the American Chemical Society. 2001;**123**:8628-8629

[3] Aime S, Barge A, Delli Castelli D, Fedeli F, Mortillaro A, Nielsen FU, Terreno E. Paramagnetic lanthanide (III) complexes as pH-sensitive chemical exchange saturation transfer (CEST) contrast agents for MRI applications. Magnetic Resonance in Medicine. 2002; **47**:639-648

[4] Snoussi K, Bulte JWM, Gueron M, van Zijl PCM. Sensitive CEST agents based on nucleic acid imino proton exchange: Detection of poly(rU) and of a dendrimer-poly(rU) model for nucleic acid delivery and pharmacology. Magnetic Resonance in Medicine. 2003;**49**: 998-1005

[5] Zhou J, Lal B, Wilson DA, Laterra J, van Zijl PCM. Amide proton transfer (APT) contrast for imaging of brain tumors. Magnetic Resonance in Medicine. 2003;**50**:1120-1126

[6] Sun PZ, Murata Y, Lu J, Wang X, Lo EH, Sorensen AG. Relaxation-compensated fast multislice amide proton transfer (APT) imaging of acute ischemic stroke. Magnetic Resonance in Medicine. 2008;**59**:1175-1182

[7] Harris RJ, Cloughesy TF, Liau LM, Prins RM, Antonios JP, Li D, Yong WH, Pope WB, Lai A, Nghiemphu PL, Ellingson BM. pH-weighted molecular imaging of gliomas using amine chemical exchange saturation transfer MRI. Neuro Oncol. 2015;**17**:1514-1524

[8] Van Zijl PCM, Jones CK, Ren J, Malloy CR, Sherry AD. MRI detection of glycogen *in vivo* by using chemical exchange saturation transfer imaging (glycoCEST). Proceedings of the National Academy of Sciences of the United States of America. 2007;**104**:4359-4364

[9] Ling W, Regatte RR, Navon G, Jerschow A. Assessment of glycosaminoglycan concentration in vivo by chemical exchange-dependent saturation transfer (gagCEST). Proceedings of the National Academy of Sciences of the United States of America. 2008;**105**: 2266-2270

[10] Cai K, Haris M, Singh A, Kogan F, Greenberg JH, Hariharan H, Detre JA, Reddy R. Magnetic resonance imaging of glutamate. Nature Medicine. 2012;**18**:302-306

[11] Jones KM, Pollard AC, Pagel MD. Clinical applications of chemical exchange saturation transfer (CEST) MRI. Journal of Magnetic Resonance Imaging. 2017 (in press)

[12] Walker-Samuel S, Ramasawmy R, Torrealdea F, Rega M, Rajkumar V, Johnson SP, Richardson S, Gonçalves M, Parkes HG, Arstad E, Thomas DL, Pedley RB, Lythgoe MF, Golay X. In vivo imaging of glucose uptake and metabolism in tumors. Nature Medicine. 2013;**19**:1067-1072

[13] Chen LQ, Howison CM, Jeffery JJ, Robey IF, Kuo PH, Pagel MD. Evaluations of extracellular pH within in vivo tumors using acidoCEST MRI. Magnetic Resonance in Medicine. 2014;**72**:1408-1417

[14] Maruyama S, Ueda J, Kimura A, Murase K. Development and characterization of novel LipoCEST agents based on thermosensitive liposomes. Magnetic Resonance in Medical Sciences. 2016;**15**:324-334

[15] Sun PZ. Simultaneous determination of labile proton concentration and exchange rate utilizing optimal RF power: Radio frequency power (RFP) dependence of chemical exchange saturation transfer (CEST) MRI. Journal of Magnetic Resonance. 2010;**202**: 155-161

[16] Sun PZ. Simplified and scalable numerical solution for describing multi-pool chemical exchange saturation transfer (CEST) MRI contrast. Journal of Magnetic Resonance. 2010;**205**: 235-241

[17] Woessner DE, Zhang S, Merritt ME, Sherry AD. Numerical solution of the Bloch equations provides insights into the optimum design of PARACEST agents for MRI. Magnetic Resonance in Medicine. 2005;**53**:790-799

[18] Murase K, Tanki N. Numerical solutions to the time-dependent Bloch equations revisited. Magnetic Resonance Imaging. 2011;**29**:126-131

[19] Koss H, Rance M, Palmer AG. General expression for $R_{1\rho}$ relaxation for *N*-site chemical exchange and the special case of linear chains. Journal of Magnetic Resonance. 2017;**274**:36-45

[20] Murase K. Numerical analysis of the magnetization behavior in magnetic resonance imaging in the presence of multiple chemical exchange pools. Open Journal of Applied Sciences. 2017;**7**:1-14

[21] Mulkern RV, Williams ML. The general solution to the Bloch equation with constant rf and relaxation terms: Application to saturation and slice selection. Medical Physics. 1993;**20**:5-13

[22] Murase K. A theoretical and numerical consideration of the longitudinal and transverse relaxations in the rotating frame. Magnetic Resonance Imaging. 2013;**31**:1544-1558

[23] Li X, Han ET, Busse RF, Majumdar S. *In vivo* $T_{1}\rho$ mapping in cartilage using 3D magnetization prepared angle-modulated partitioned *k*-space spoiled gradient echo snapshots (3D MAPSS). Magnetic Resonance in Medicine. 2008;**59**:298-307

[24] Regatte RR, Akella SV, Borthakur A, Kneeland JB, Reddy R. *In vivo* proton MR three-dimensional $T_{1}\rho$ mapping of human articular cartilage: Initial experience. Radiology. 2003;**229**:269-274

[25] Santyr GE, Henkelman RM, Bronskill MJ. Spin locking for magnetic resonance imaging with application to human breast. Magnetic Resonance in Medicine. 1989;**12**:25-37

[26] Markkola AT, Aronen HJ, Paavonen T, Hopsu E, Sipila LM, Tanttu JI, Sepponen RE. Spin lock and magnetization transfer imaging of head and neck tumors. Radiology. 1996;**200**:369-375

[27] Jin T, Autio J, Obata T, Kim S-G. Spin-locking versus chemical exchange saturation transfer MRI for investigating chemical exchange process between water and labile metabolite protons. Magnetic Resonance in Medicine. 2011;**65**:1448-1460

[28] Kogan F, Singh A, Cai K, Haris M, Hariharan H, Reddy R. Investigation of chemical exchange at intermediate exchange rates using a combination of chemical exchange saturation transfer (CEST) and spin-locking methods (CESTrho). Magnetic Resonance in Medicine. 2012;**68**:107-119

[29] Trott O, Palmer AG. $R1\rho$ relaxation outside of the fast-exchange limit. Journal of Magnetic Resonance. 2002;**154**:157-160

[30] Murase K. Behavior of the magnetization in spin-locking magnetic resonance imaging using numerical solutions to the time-dependent Bloch equations. Physics in Medicine and Biology. 2012;**57**:N481-N492

[31] Nelder JA, Mead R. A simplex method for function minimization. The Computer Journal. 1965;**7**:308-313

[32] Sun PZ, Zhou J, Huang J, van Zijl P. Simplified quantitative description of amide proton transfer (APT) imaging during acute ischemia. Magnetic Resonance in Medicine. 2007;**57**: 405-410

[33] Trott O, Palmer AG. Theoretical study of $R_{1\rho}$ rotating-frame and R_2 free-precession relaxation in the presence of n-site chemical exchange. Journal of Magnetic Resonance. 2004;**170**:104-112

[34] Grey MJ, Wang C, Palmer AG. Disulfide bond isomerization in basic pancreatic trypsin inhibitor: Multisite chemical exchange quantified by CPMG relaxation dispersion and chemical shift modeling. Journal of the American Chemical Society. 2003;**125**:14324-14335

[35] Ji Y, Zhou IY, Qiu B, Sun PZ. Progress toward quantitative in vivo chemical exchange saturation transfer (CEST) MRI. Israel Journal of Chemistry. 2017;**57**:1-17

[36] Padormoa F, Beqiria A, Hajnalab JV, Malika SJ. Parallel transmission for ultrahigh-field imaging. NMR in Biomedicine. 2016;**29**:1145-1161

[37] Kim M, Gillen J, Landman BA, Zhou J, Van Zijl PC. Water saturation shift referencing (WASSR) for chemical exchange saturation transfer (CEST) experiments. Magnetic Resonance in Medicine. 2009;**61**:1441-1450

[38] Zhou J, Blakeley JO, Hua J, Kim M, Laterra J, Pomper MG, Van Zijl PC. Practical data acquisition method for human brain tumor amide proton transfer (APT) imaging. Magnetic Resonance in Medicine. 2008;**60**:842-849

[39] Singh A, Cai K, Haris M, Hariharan H, Reddy R. On B_1 Inhomogeneity correction of *in vivo* human brain glutamate chemical exchange saturation transfer contrast at 7T. Magnetic Resonance in Medicine. 2013;**69**:818-824

[40] Windschuh J, Zaiss M, Meissner J-E, Paech D, Radbruch A, Ladd ME, Bachert P. Correction of B_1-inhomogeneities for relaxation-compensated CEST imaging at 7T. NMR in Biomedicine. 2015;**28**:529-537

[41] Schuenke P, Windschuh J, Roeloffs V, Ladd ME, Bachert P, Zaiss M. Simultaneous mapping of water shift and B_1 (WASABI)-application to field-inhomogeneity correction of CEST MRI data. Magnetic Resonance in Medicine. 2017;**77**:571-580

[42] Sun PZ, Farrar CT, Sorensen AG. Correction for artifacts induced by B_0 and B_1 field inhomogeneities in pH-sensitive chemical exchange saturation transfer (CEST) imaging. Magnetic Resonance in Medicine. 2007;**58**:1207-1215